Sports Medicine for Coaches and Athletes

SOCCER

Sports Medicine for Coaches and Athletes

A series edited by Adil E. Shamoo, University of Maryland School of Medicine at Baltimore, USA

This series of monographs is devoted to the application of sports medicine research to specific sports. It is intended to present current medical information in a succinct format that is understandable and practical for participants and others directly involved in the individual sports.

Volume 1
Sports Medicine for Coaches and Athletes — Soccer
Adil E. Shamoo, William H. Baugher, and *Robert M. Germeroth*

Additional volumes forthcoming

Sports Medicine for Coaches and Athletes — Basketball

Sports Medicine for Coaches and Athletes — Football

This book is part of a series. The publisher will accept continuation orders which may be cancelled at any time and which provide for automatic billing and shipping of each title in the series upon publication. Please write for details.

Sports Medicine for Coaches And Athletes

SOCCER

Adil E. Shamoo, PhD

*University of Maryland School of Medicine
at Baltimore*

William H. Baugher, MD

Sports Medicine Orthopedist

Robert M. Germeroth, PT

*Bennett Institute for Sports Medicine
and Rehabilitation
Baltimore, Maryland*

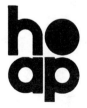 **harwood academic publishers**

Australia • Austria • China • France • Germany •
India • Japan • Luxembourg • Malaysia •
Netherlands • Russia • Singapore • Switzerland •
Thailand • United Kingdom • United States

Copyright © 1995 by Harwood Academic Publishers GmbH.

3 Boulevard Royal
L-2449 Luxembourg

British Library Cataloguing in Publication Data

Shamoo, Adil E.
  Soccer. – (Sports Medicine for Coaches &
  Athletes Series; Vol. 1)
  I. Title II. Series
  613.711

  ISBN   3-7186-0600-3   (hardcover)
          3-7186-0601-1   (softcover)

To

Abe, Zach, and Jessica
Susan and William
Jessica and Julie

CONTENTS

INTRODUCTION TO THE SERIES

The science of sports medicine and exercise physiology is expanding rapidly. However, this growing body of knowledge is becoming increasingly complex and is not easily accessible to the athletes, coaches, trainers, and sports enthusiasts in most need of this material. The *Sports Medicine for Coaches and Athletes* series is designed to explain the scientific basis of athletic performance by translating complex scientific data into general, practical information and by providing training, nutritional, and injury prevention and treatment guidelines that are specific for each individual or team sport.

Adil E. Shamoo, PhD

FOREWORD

Should players drink only a few sips of water before a game to make sure their stomachs are not "weighted down"? Is water the best drink during a game, or are "sports drinks" better?

You will find the answers in this book, which fills a definite niche in the soccer coach's library.

Most books on coaching soccer mention injuries; some have a chapter on the subject; here is a unique volume dedicated to the subject of soccer injuries, their prevention and treatment.

The first chapter highlights the criteria for optimal performance, which helps the coach decide what makes a good soccer player, and deals with all aspects of the complete player — physical, mental, social, and psychological. Most coaches will find this helpful in selecting their competitive teams.

Some readers might tend to skip the next two chapters, which give the theory behind the principles laid down in the rest of the book. However, even if you are not interested in the biochemical and physiological reasons for the practices recommended in the treatment section, these chapters lay the foundation for understanding why one treatment is better than another.

Chapter 4 gives clear, practical advice on dealing with injuries and will help the coach decide when an injury is beyond his/her ability to administer treatment.

The remainder of the volume provides invaluable information about the effects of nutrition, water, sports drinks, and other substances on the soccer player.

Finally, chapter 9 offers those of us who coach young women some insights as to when and how their training should differ from that of young men. It is now becoming apparent the approach to coaching girls should be different from that used in coaching boys; this book continues that discourse and extends the understanding of this phenomenon.

The Soccer Association of Columbia is happy to have Adil Shamoo, who is one of the authors, as one of our coaches and recommends that soccer coaches pay serious attention to this book.

Gregory Dash
President
Soccer Association of Columbia
Columbia, Maryland

PREFACE

In the past twenty years, there has been an increased interest among American youth in playing soccer or, as the rest of the world calls it, football. Also, there has been advancement in fundamental scientific knowledge relating to sports and exercise physiology, adaptation, and medicine, as reflected in the greater number of articles and books on these subjects. However, this information tends to be general and not readily digested by or directly relevant to soccer players, coaches, and parents. At times, even physicians, whether pediatricians, internists, or orthopedists, find it difficult to translate current knowledge into practice. Soccer players and coaches represent a new breed of highly motivated individuals eager to do their best for the game. Their lack of background knowledge, however, precludes them from utilizing scientific research accumulated recently in sports medicine for practical use on and off the field. Up-to-date information would help prepare coach and athlete for better results in terms of prevention of injury, better training, adaptation, proper course of action before, during and after the game, proper rehabilitation, and knowing when to consult a trainer or physician. Current research could help to win more games in an enjoyable environment.

We wrote this book because of our strong belief that there was a great need for it; we also wanted to serve the soccer community. Because each of us brings his own perspective to the text, this monograph is a unique compilation of ideas, facts, and figures. Adil E. Shamoo has been playing, coaching, and observing soccer for years; in addition, he teaches sports medicine. William H. Baugher is a practicing orthopedist dealing with large numbers of soccer players with various injuries ranging from superficial to serious. Robert M. Germeroth is a physical therapist treating soccer players' injuries, overseeing their rehabilitation, and, more importantly, advising them on proper conditioning. This book is written with players and coaches in mind. The presentation ranges from the very simple to the complex, so that players, coaches, and parents can trace treatment to the scientific logic and reasoning behind the procedure. It is hoped that more sophisticated readers will delve further into the subject.

The authors wish to thank Leonard P. Kapcala, MD, associate professor at the University of Maryland School of Medicine, for critically reviewing the manuscript. He is an avid soccer fan, player, and, occasionally, a coach.

To our knowledge, this is the first monograph of its kind. Therefore, we are certain we may have omitted several aspects of soccer and included others that were not pertinent. In all sincerity, we welcome readers' suggestions, criticisms, and corrections. We plan to revise the text whenever feasible. Please write to Adil E. Shamoo, PhD, Department of Biological Chemistry, University of Maryland School of Medicine, 108 N. Greene Street, Baltimore, Maryland 21201-1503, USA.

ABOUT THE AUTHORS

ADIL E. SHAMOO, PhD
Professor and former chairman of the Department of Biological Chemistry, University of Maryland School of Medicine in Baltimore (1977–present). Formerly at the University of Rochester School of Medicine in New York (1973–1979), he also served one year (1972–1973) at the National Institutes of Health. Dr. Shamoo obtained his PhD in Biophysics in 1970 from the City University of New York. His research for the past twenty years has been in the area of biochemistry and biophysics of the skeletal and cardiac muscles. More recently, Dr. Shamoo has been studying the effects of dopamine, a brain neurotransmitter. He has contributed to more than 150 research papers. In addition, Dr. Shamoo has edited books and journals, and he has chaired numerous international conferences. He is a member of a large number of professional organizations, as well as having held leadership positions, and is a member of the American College of Sports Medicine. Dr. Shamoo has given more than 150 lectures worldwide on various topics.

Dr. Shamoo played soccer as a youngster and has been coaching since 1979. He has coached neighborhood teams, travel teams (boys and girls), and was assistant to a high school coach (1989–1991). He was travel team coordinator for the Soccer Association of Columbia (SAC) (1985–1987). Dr. Shamoo holds a USSF referee license class I (1986) and USSF coaching licenses D (1982) and C (1989), and he has lectured widely to coaches on sports medicine. He has been teaching an elective course to medical students on the "Biochemical Basis of Sports Medicine" since 1986.

WILLIAM H. BAUGHER, MD
Currently in private practice as a sports medicine orthopedist of a large sports medicine practice group in Baltimore,

Maryland. He is a member of active and visiting staff of several hospitals, including University of Maryland Hospital, Union Memorial Hospital, and Johns Hopkins Hospital. Dr. Baugher was formerly at the University of Maryland School of Medicine, Division of Orthopedics; and Johns Hopkins School of Medicine, Division of Orthopedic–Sports Medicine. He is a former fellow in orthopedic–sports medicine at The Hospital for Special Surgery–Cornell University Medical College, in New York City.

Dr. Baugher completed his medical education in 1972 at Charlottesville, Virginia, and his internship and residency at Washington University in Saint Louis, Missouri. He was chief resident (1977–1978) at the University of Virginia Medical Center, Charlottesville, Virginia.

Dr. Baugher has published and lectured widely in the field of sports medicine especially as it relates to hand, wrist, and knee injuries. He has been certified by the American Board of Orthopedic Surgery since 1981, with an added certificate of qualifications in hand surgery since 1990. Dr. Baugher is a member of the American Academy of Orthopedic Surgeons, the American Society for Surgery of the Hand, and the American Orthopedic Society for Sports Medicine.

ROBERT M. GERMEROTH, PT, MBA

Director of Sports Medicine at the Bennett Institute for Sports Medicine and Rehabilitation since 1983, a program of Children's Hospital in Baltimore, Maryland. This is one of the largest sports medicine organizations in the geographic area. He received a degree in physical therapy in 1978 from the University of Maryland at Baltimore and a Master's in Business Administration in 1988 from the University of Baltimore. Mr. Germeroth has been a consultant to the Baltimore Orioles and the Baltimore Thunder; and a large part of his practice deals with soccer injuries. He has made numerous presentations to physicians, athletic trainers, and therapists on the subject of sports medicine and orthopedics, and is a member of the American Physical Therapy Association (APTA), the Sports Medicine and Orthopedic sections of APTA, and the National Youth Sports Foundation.

Chapter

ONE

Criteria for Optimal Performance

Soccer is a major sport for young athletes in the United States, and is also rapidly becoming a major sport for males and females of all ages. Because young athletes go through puberty at different times, there is a great deal of variation among these athletes in terms of size and maturity. These differences pose a challenge to the athletes and to their coaches. The primary characteristics of a young athlete are: motivation; physical fitness (i.e., muscle strength, power, endurance, flexibility, proper body composition, and cardiorespiratory endurance); discipline; coachability; skills; ability to be a part of a team; ability to think under stress; and good spatial orientation. Soccer practice sessions should seek to achieve physical conditioning, repetitive training, a proper intensity of training, flexibility, and the awareness that the achievement of proper endurance for the soccer athlete requires at least 4–6 months of training. Also, the coach should be aware that extreme and severe high intensity and high frequency training causes damage to muscle tissues and is counterproductive to the goals of the athlete.

We will restrict this section to discussing training as it relates to soccer. Several of the statements in this section will be expanded upon in subsequent chapters.

Soccer has become a major youth sport in the United States. It is estimated that over 15 million youngsters play soccer at various levels. Soccer is not thought of as a contact sport; however, body contact does occur as part of the normal flow of play. Although injuries due to soccer are relatively low compared to other sports, for those above 18 years old the injury rate is about 6–8%. Most injuries for those below 12 years of age occur in the lower extremities due to blows to these regions or due to overuse and improper training. Most injuries in soccer occur at the ankle, foot, knee, and skin. Less frequent injuries occur in the abdomen, head, and neck. Goalies tend to have more injuries. Female soccer players tend to have higher rates of injuries than males.

BENEFITS OF PLAYING SOCCER

The benefits of playing soccer for youngsters and adults are similar to those of other sports that require repeated physical exercise. In general, sports improve the quality of life because of the benefits to one's health. More specifically, playing soccer increases muscle strength, endurance, and flexibility. Moreover, soccer enhances cardiovascular endurance, contributes to the prevention of illnesses, enhances self-esteem, improves stress management and it is true recreation and fun. To some, playing soccer may become a lifelong form of exercise and enjoyment.

PHYSIOLOGICAL AND CHRONOLOGICAL AGE

All middle school teachers can tell you that adolescent teenagers are difficult to handle and that they vary a great deal in size, height, and their level of maturity. This is because teen-agers, in addition to possessing the normal genetic inheritance of size from their parents, are also in a very fast growth period (puberty), especially during the growth spurt. On the average, the growth spurt occurs around 12 years of age for girls and 14 years of age for boys. Because of these changes, young athletes are experiencing a tumultuous period which affects them both physiologically and hormonally. Therefore, young athletes of the same age group who play soccer are very different in terms of size, shape, height, and skill level. Because of these differen-ces, it is very difficult to mold the players of this age group into a cohesive team.

SELECTION OF PLAYERS

There are basically two types of young soccer teams: neighbor-hood teams and travel teams (select teams). In addition, high schools have varsity and junior varsity soccer teams. Some middle schools also have soccer teams.

In neighborhood teams, everyone can register and play for their approximate age group. Usually, neighborhood teams span an age bracket of one or two years in order to have a sufficient number of players. In addition, there is either no selection process or a simple mechanism of scoring players based on simple skills and physical abilities. Because of the two year age bracket and different growth spurts among the young players, they tend to be very heterogeneous in terms of skill, speed, and sizes. Such a mix represents a greater risk for in-juries as well as frustrations for the youngster, particularly if the coach is very demanding. The composition of the team presents a greater problem to the coach in terms of all of the training factors which will be discussed later.

The select teams usually span a one year age bracket. The level of skill is better than that of neighborhood teams. How-ever, despite the one year bracket between the ages, the team still varies a great deal in sizes and skill levels. Usually, because of puberty such teams are dominated by tall, fast, and large players. These differences become insignificant as players pass puberty. One suggestion for young teams consisting of players below 14 years of age is to determine teams based not only on the players' age but also on their height and weight as is the case in football. However, because there is much less physical contact in soccer than in football, grouping by weight is not as critical in soccer.

CHARACTERISTICS OF A SOCCER PLAYER

All of the following player characteristics need not be present before the individual plays soccer. However, the individual should either show aptitude or at least a willingness to acquire these characteristics.

1. **Motivation**. The soccer player should be interested and motivated to play the game of soccer (i.e., kicking a ball, running, passing a ball etc). In other words, the player should get enjoyment out of performing these tasks, especially when these tasks are performed spontaneously and without pressure from adults.

2. **Physical Fitness**. The term physical fitness connotes different meanings for different activities. In the context of soccer, it is the ability to play soccer for 60–90 minutes without fatigue, exhaustion, or other symptoms that interfere with performance. The player should have the following physical fitness characteristics to play soccer: a) muscle strength and power; b) endurance; c) flexibility; d) proper body composition; e) cardiac respiratory endurance; f) coordination.

3. **Discipline**. The player should have the ability to practice and play the game in a repeated fashion several times a week.

4. **Coachability**. The player should have the ability to accept instructions and to try to comply with these instructions.

5. **Skills or the ability to learn skills**. The player should have the ability to conduct or learn individual soccer skills with the ball such as kicking, receiving, passing, shooting, control, etc.

6. **Ability to play in a team sport**. This describes the ability of the player to cooperate with other team members to achieve a difficult task. Also, the player should be able to sacrifice personal recognition for the sake of the team. The player also should be able to associate with others for prolonged periods of

time and sometimes under stressful conditions. Finally, the player should have the ability to enjoy himself with others.

7. **Ability to think under stress.** Most people are not as logical under stressful conditions as they are normally. However, the well trained soccer player learns what to do under the various game conditions, and also learns to think quickly under stressful conditions.

8. **Proper spatial orientation.** The ability to think and visualize in three dimensions with respect to the soccer field is difficult for very young players. The player should be able to learn to adapt to the spatial orientation within the field and reposition himself/herself relevant to the ball, teammates, and opposing team members.

STEPS TO PLAYING SOCCER

Figure 1.1 is a schematic diagram of the steps needed to be undertaken to prepare a soccer player for the season.

PRACTICE SESSIONS

The purpose of this monograph is not to suggest specific exercises. There are other sources addressing various exercises/drills which pertain to soccer practice session. However, we will give a general outline that all soccer practice sessions should include. In this manner, coaches can use their creativity to make soccer practices more enjoyable and more beneficial to the different needs of the varied groups.

The practice sessions should be designed to make the individual a better soccer player. The best practice for any sport is to play that sport repeatedly in order to develop those muscles, skills, endurance, etc., for that sport. It is common for those who play one sport and then suddenly play another sport to have muscle aches after the first few times of participation in the new sport. The muscle aches are usually due to the use of the same muscle in a different way and frequently a different set of muscle fibers than those used before. This is known as "specificity of training." Thus, the more the soccer player plays soccer, the better he/she will become in soccer. This is not to say

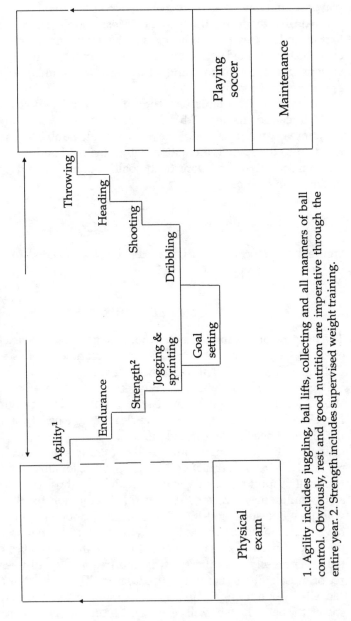

Training for 3–6 months to develop abilities in:

Agility[1]
Endurance
Strength[2]
Jogging & sprinting
Goal setting
Dribbling
Shooting
Heading
Throwing

Playing soccer

Maintenance

Physical exam

1. Agility includes juggling, ball lifts, collecting and all manners of ball control. Obviously, rest and good nutrition are imperative through the entire year. 2. Strength includes supervised weight training.

Figure 1.1. Steps to playing soccer.

that the game of soccer should not be broken down into small segments so that it can be taught and repeatedly reinforced.

In order to prepare the individual to play soccer, players and coaches should observe the following factors:

1. **Physical conditioning**. This involves the increased ability to sustain both aerobic and anaerobic exercises.

2. **Frequency of training**. This should be 2–3 times a week for youngsters and 3–4 times a week for adults.

3. **Intensity of training**. During a 60–90 minute exercise session there should be periods (1–3) lasting at least 15 minutes long (for optimal adaptation) wherein the player's oxygen consumption (in liters per minutes) should be at about 70% of VO_{2max}. However, the range of intensity of exercise can be from 40 to 70% (i.e., 55 to 80% increase in heart rate). The VO_{2max} is the maximal oxygen uptake by an individual due to an increase in workload (e.g., pedaling a bicycle with increased resistance to rotation of the wheel while measuring oxygen consumption). This translates into about an 80–90% increase in heart rate (i.e., about 140–150 beats/min). This is the best way to induce muscle and cardio-respiratory endurance. However, most soccer players, especially young players, can practice at suboptimal levels of intensity for adaptation. The suboptimal level of practice simply would lengthen the time needed to reach optimal adaptation.

4. **Flexibility exercises**. The full range of motion of muscles, joints, tendons, and ligaments is important to maintain proper function for soccer and also to prevent injury to these sites. As a result of years of "personal observation" of soccer players of all ages (this observation may not be universal), it is apparent that even some elite players have inadequate flexibility. This is probably a reflection of limited emphasis on flexibility exercises by the coaches rather than the inherent poor flexibility of the soccer player. Because muscle temperature in extremities is slightly lower than core temperature, increased circulation of blood into the muscle during exercise helps the muscle to function optimally. In addition, flexibility exercises help prevent deleterious effects due to ischemia (i.e., inadequate blood flow). Therefore, it is important that the athlete warms up by individual skill exercises or jogging (not sprinting) one or two laps around the field before stretching. Stretching exercises

without proper warm-up could cause pulled muscles and other injuries. Furthermore, stretching should be static (stretching gradually to full range) and not ballistic (quick extension of arms, legs and other parts of the body). Ballistic stretching could cause injury, especially under poor warm-up conditions. Static stretching should last 10–30 seconds and be repeated 3–5 times. Each stretching exercise should include a larger range of motion than the previous one. Stretching can also be achieved during the practice. In addition, after each rigorous practice session, there should be 10 minutes of low to moderate cool down exercises. Examples of cool down exercises in soccer are individual skill exercises, light jogging, and perhaps best of all, just walking or dribbling the ball lightly (for further details see Chapter 3).

   5. **Time to peak endurance.** Quick and strenuous training for 2–3 weeks prior to a season (as is the case in some high schools after a sedentary summer) cannot achieve endurance and may be detrimental to the athlete. This is because adaptation of the cardiorespiratory system and muscle enzymes requires about six months of training to reach peak endurance capacity. However, psychological training could improve performance without additional muscular adaptation. Moreover, it takes 2–4 weeks without training (as may be the case during the summer for high schoolers) to lose most endurance parameters (see Chapter 6 on endurance for details).

   Therefore, a well planned training period is an essential part of preparing players for the season. In an ideal situation, year round training is highly recommended.

SUGGESTED PRACTICE SESSION

Figure 1.2 represents an example of a single week long soccer practice session. All muscles used in soccer should be warmed and stretched. Main areas of concern are: upper leg (groin, hamstrings, quads), abdominals, back, ankles, and neck. The practice session should start with a warm-up (Wu) including quick paced individual soccer skills, dribbling, or jogging 1–2 laps around the field, followed by stretching exercises. After Wu the team should be broken into 2–4 groups, each practicing

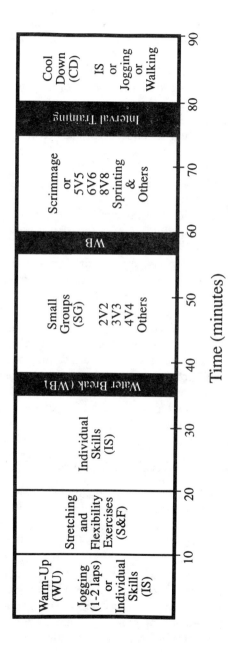

Figure 1.2. Example of activities for a 90-minute practice session for young soccer players.

different individual skills. The number of water breaks should be increased from the suggested 2 breaks to 4; in addition, practice may be canceled if the weather is too hot and humid. Individual skill practice is followed by small group practices composed of any combination of 2V2, 3V3, 4V4, or other similar practices in a small field (i.e., 1/6th to 1/8th of a soccer field), in order to provide frequent contact with the ball by each player. In fact, young athletes, especially those below 12 years of age, should play their games on a field half the size of the regulation field. Regulation fields have widths which range from a minimum of 50 yards to a maximum of 100 yards, and lengths which range from a minimum of 100 yards to a maximum of 130 yards. It is not necessary to have an actual scrimmage each practice; for example, at times team scrimmages can be substituted with smaller scrimmages composed of 6V6, 8V8, etc. The drills can be followed by a short interval training whereby the athlete sprints and rests for increasing lengths of time. For example, the players can sprint from the goal line to 18, 20, 50, 80, and 100 yards with a rest period of about 15 sec to 1 min between each run. Of course, the length of interval training depends on the physical fitness of the players. Finally, in the last ten minutes of the practice session there should be a cool down period consisting of moderate exercises such as practicing ball skills, dribbling the ball, stretching or simply fast paced walking. Only the last and first two parts of every practice session should remain constant.

MUSCLE STRENGTH AND POWER

In general, young athletes should not engage in weight lifting exercises. However, the use of moderate weight lifting for young athletes in order to moderately increase their strength and power is an acceptable form of exercise under the strict supervision of a strength training specialist. The strict supervision of weight bearing exercises for young athletes is important to prevent the occurrence of serious injury. For example, children below 13 years of age should not perform weight bearing exercises in the standing position where there is a great deal of compression force on the legs. In order to increase muscle strength, the muscle should be challenged by at least 60% of the maximal weight lifted the first time. Furthermore, in subsequent days and weeks, the muscle must be challenged by increasing weights, with low repetition (e.g., 10 times) or lower weight with high frequency repetition (up to 15). Remember, an increase in muscle strength is not necessarily associated with a large increase in muscle size. Strength training with low frequency repetition increases the size of the muscle (body building) but not necessarily muscle strength. While defenders may be able to use a greater muscle mass and strength, other soccer players need to increase strength more than muscle size in order to maintain their agility and speed.

PRE-GAME MEALS

A few days before a single soccer game, there is no need for a special diet if the player has been eating balanced meals. Glycogen loading (eating large amounts of carbohydrate 2–3 days before the event followed by rest the day before the event) is not needed for most soccer games; however, glycogen loading can be advantageous for events lasting over 90 minutes (e.g., marathon running) where glycogen storage becomes a rate limiting factor for energy supply. Soccer players rarely run continuously for 90 minutes in a single game. However, when there is a weekend tournament where 3–5 games are played in 3 days, moderate glycogen loading is acceptable.

Pre-game meals should be scheduled no less than 2–4 hours before the game. The closer the meal time is to the game, the lighter the meal should be, and the more liquid in nature. In any case, in all pre-game meals, the player should avoid fats and proteins. Carbohydrates, which are prevalent in foods such as pancakes and spaghetti are more appropriate choices. In addition, the athlete should avoid sweet foods just prior to the event (up to 1 hr before the game) to avoid increased insulin secretion (hyperinsulinemia) which could possibly result in lower than normal blood glucose levels (hypoglycemia). Insulin is a hormone that regulates the levels of sugar in blood. The resulting hyperinsulinemia and thus low blood sugar is thought to be associated with poor exercise performance. However, during exercise, ingestion of glucose does not result in increased insulin secretion because of increased catecholamine secretion (hormones such as norepinephrine and epinephrine) which suppresses insulin secretion. In addition, before game time the player should drink 1–2 glasses of cold water to insure proper hydration.

During the game, the athlete should drink only cold water, especially on hot and humid days. However, regardless of the environment, cold water should be utilized in amounts greater than the thirst requirement. For every 1 pound lost during practice or a game, the athlete should drink 1 large glass of water (400–500 ml). In one soccer game per day, drinking liquid carbohydrates may be unnecessary for young people. However, for a soccer player in a professional game drinking liquid carbohydrates (or polymers) just before or during the game may be useful. The ingestion of liquid food during the game may retard hydration of the body from the ingestion of pure cold water.

POST-GAME

After the game, it is recommended that the player should rest, drink water and juices, and eat vegetables and well balanced meals. Close attention to the proper foods will benefit the individual for the next practice and game. If after a game, persistent headaches or dizziness occurs, the athlete should see his/her physician.

HEAVY TRAINING

Fortunately, few soccer coaches resort to very heavy schedules in terms of both the frequency and intensity (e.g., 5 times a week, 4–5 hours per day, with strenuous exercises and high intensity training) of training. Some coaches keep the intensity of training so high that players may collapse from exhaustion. This type of training is not only detrimental to the individual's well being but also counterproductive to the coach's stated goals. During exercise, muscle protein synthesis is suppressed. Strenuous exercise has been shown to increase the level of muscle enzymes and proteins in the blood, which is indicative of muscle tissue damage. This is because the damaged cells in muscle tissue leak their contents (i.e., enzymes and proteins) to the capillaries and eventually these proteins appear in the blood. This is similar to finding heart muscle enzymes and proteins in the blood after a heart attack. Moreover, severe training could result in the appearance of red blood cells and other blood constituents in urine. This is because of extreme high hydrostatic pressure exerted on kidney blood flow.

FURTHER GENERAL READING

Hong, C.Z., and Lien, I. (1984). Metabolic Effects of Exhaustive Training of Athletes, *Arch. Phys. Med. Rehabil.* 65:362–365.

Dohm, G.L., et al. (1987). Protein Metabolism During Endurance Exercise, *Fed. Proc.* 44:348–352.

Kibler, W.B. (1993). Injuries in Adolescent and Preadolescent Soccer Players. *Med. Sci. Sports Exerc.* 25:1330–1332.

Chapter

TWO

Types of Training for Soccer

The ultimate source of energy for the body is adenosine triphosphate (ATP). The immediate replenishing source of ATP is phosphocreatine phosphate (PCr). However, ATP and PCr combined will only sustain energy for less than 10 seconds in an exhaustive exercise. Food is processed either through glycolysis (in this process oxygen (O_2) is not utilized; i.e., it is an "anaerobic" process) to yield a quick but yet inefficient source of ATP, or through oxidation (here, O_2 is utilized; i.e., oxidation is an "aerobic" process) which yields a slow and very efficient source of ATP. The anaerobic process produces lactate which contributes to fatigue. Soccer is a mixture of aerobic and anaerobic exercise. Therefore, the athlete should train via a combination of sprint-like exercises, jogging, and running to adapt to both types of exercises.

ENERGY SOURCE

The immediate source of energy for muscle activity within each cell is adenosine triphosphate (ATP). Muscle action is an organized composite of the action of individual cells. ATP is an intracellular substance which contains three phosphate molecules, and it is through the breakdown of the terminal phosphate that energy is produced. The amount of ATP available in each cell is very small, and only provides sufficient energy to last less than 1–2 seconds in an exhaustive sprint-like exercise. However, the cell attempts to maintain a fairly constant level of ATP, especially during moderate activities. The protein which helps to provide an immediate source of ATP is the molecule phosphocreatine phosphate (PCr). PCr phosphorylates (i.e., adds one phosphate) adenosine diphosphate (ADP) to form ATP. The amount of ATP and PCr combined however, lasts less than about 10 seconds in an exhaustive exercise. The long range source of energy for the cell comes from two main processes that involve utilizing the energy stored in foodstuffs. These two processes are:

(1) **Glycolysis**. ATP is produced anaerobically (without oxygen) from sugar derived from stored muscle glycogen. Glycogen is a polysaccharide (i.e., it consists of many sugars) molecule consisting of hundreds to thousands of glucose molecules linked together. Anaerobic exercise produces lactic acid which can accumulate and have adverse effects on performance. However, the anaerobic process does provide ATP when the body needs it as a quick source of energy (i.e., for sprint-like exercise).

(2) **Oxidation**. ATP is produced aerobically (with oxygen) from carbohydrates, fats, and proteins. The aerobic oxidation process produces 13 times more ATP for the same amount of starting material than ATP which is anaerobically produced by glycolysis. While the aerobic process is slow, it provides long lasting energy for exercises such as jogging and marathon running.

Figure 2.1 gives a hypothetical order of the utilization of energy in soccer playing. Cellular ATP and ATP derived from phosphorylation by PCr are utilized first. Soccer players simultaneously use the anaerobic and the aerobic systems as the situation demands.

A well trained soccer player has an advantage over the untrained person in the utilization of energy. In Chapter 6 we describe in detail the biochemical changes due to training. However, we will briefly describe the physiological and biochemical advantages of a trained soccer player in utilizing the energy pyramid of Figure 2.1.

In a trained soccer player, the levels of ATP and PCr are higher and thus last about 20–30% longer than in an untrained player. More importantly, the trained soccer player has a greater glycolytic capacity (almost twice as much) as the untrained person. Furthermore, the aerobic system (i.e., enzymes, substrates etc.) is also more efficiently developed in the trained athlete. The trained athlete can therefore produce ATP faster for the aerobic exercises needed during the game. Above all, the trained soccer player can recover sooner from a bout of exercise because of the increased levels of enzymes, substrates and capacity to produce ATP.

LACTATE AND FATIGUE

The breakdown of ATP to produce energy results in the production of a hydrogen ion, and thus lowers the cellular pH. This intracellular change in pH eventually lowers the blood's pH. The presence of hydrogen ions is normally a signal for the respiratory system and kidneys to get rid of the excess hydrogen ions. However, under stressful conditions hydrogen ions and/or lactate can accumulate; eventually, the build up of these molecules may contribute to muscle fatigue. Trained athletes physiologically adapt in such a way which allows them to be able to perform adequately in the presence of higher lactate blood levels. Moreover, trained athletes tend to utilize and dissipate lactate better than untrained athletes. Therefore, the specificity of training for a given sport is important in adapting

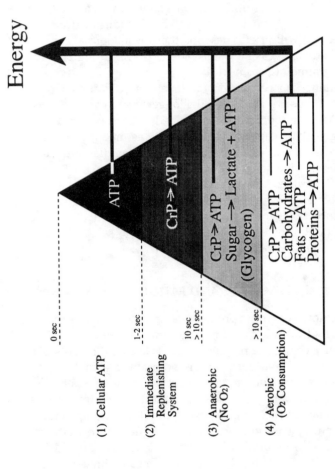

Figure 2.1. A hypothetical energy utilization pyramid for soccer players. A soccer player utilizes the needed energy from the available ATP and the quick source of ATP and the quick source of energy which is supplied by the anaerobic process — this is for when the soccer player engages in bursts of activities. The long range source of energy for soccer players is derived through aerobic processes.

the tissues to those stressful conditions of the given sport in order to stimulate cellular mechanisms of adaptation to those conditions.

After an exercise session, it is recommended that an athlete should have a cool-down period consisting of low level activities such as walking or light jogging. This cool-down period helps the blood flow through the capillaries, thus removing lactate from muscles. Rapid removal of lactate from muscles may contribute to the reduction of fatigue. Athletes also may use hot baths or saunas to enhance blood flow to muscles after an exercise session; however, this process is not recommended for players whose muscles are cramped or injured.

SOCCER AND OXYGEN UTILIZATION

In a youth soccer game, the player may run 3 to 5 miles, while in a professional soccer game the player may run 6 to 7 miles. Soccer is a mixture of aerobic (about 90% of the distance covered) and anaerobic exercise (about 10%). Therefore, the training session should combine both modalities. Aerobic (such as marathon running, jogging, etc.) sessions are usually composed of slow rhythmic exercises. These exercises allow the body to utilize oxygen to burn foodstuffs producing the required energy. Therefore, the optimal soccer training sessions should resemble match-like conditions which involve both anaerobic and aerobic exercises. These conditions consist of the player performing the following tasks:

(a) Aerobic exercises such as continuous jogging with the ball (lasting 1–5 minutes) to relocate to a new position. Repetition of this action 10–30 times per practice session.

(b) Anaerobic exercises such as sprinting, lasting from a second to 1 min. Repetition of this action 10–30 times per practice session.

Specialized players need to be cognizant of the fact that:

(a) Midfielders do most of the jogging and sprinting throughout the game because they must perform offensive and defensive tasks.

(b) Young defenders (i.e., high schools and below) tend to do more jogging than sprinting. However, at college level and above defenders tend to be similar to any other position, thus they perform both aerobic and anaerobic processes.

(c) Offensive players tend to do more sprinting than other players.

The details of the sessions should be left to the creativity of the coach. A combination of various game-like situations can be used to create an enjoyable training session. These drills can be modified to stress the specific training effect most needed by the entire team or a select group of players (i.e., defense, offense, and midfielders).

Usually, young players play more than one position (i.e., offensive versus defensive position). However, as young players pass puberty, they become more specialized in a given position. Therefore, each position may require a somewhat different emphasis.

INTERVAL TRAINING

The soccer player can benefit from interval training. Interval training consists of workouts with rest intervals varying in ratios from 1:3 to 1:1 (work/rest) depending on the need and the fitness level of the individual. The work period can range from a few seconds to several minutes, and the whole cycle can be repeated 5–20 times. A short, high intensity (sprinting) workout lasting greater than 15 seconds can improve the anaerobic system when interspersed with rest periods of 30 seconds. Interval training to improve aerobic capacity can consist of ratio's of work to rest of 1:1 or 1:1.5. The exercise period can last 60–90 seconds in order to force oxygen consumption followed with a recovery period varying from 60 to 135 seconds.

CIRCUIT TRAINING

Circuit training attempts to economize the time of exercise to improve strength, power, and the cardiorespiratory system. Exercise sessions should combine resistance (lifting weights), repetition, and rest. For example, working periods involving lifting moderate weights can vary from 30–60 seconds with similar rest periods. As many as 15 stations can be included in circuit training.

Chapter

THREE

Preparations for the Soccer Season

Soccer is a physically demanding sport. To successfully participate in soccer, the athlete must obtain a high level of physical fitness in order to accomplish the aerobic, anaerobic, and physical skills required for the sport. This chapter offers a brief discussion on the ideal pre-participation physical examination and a physical fitness evaluation. Principles of training requires attention to; overload, progressiveness, specificity, frequency, and active rest.

One reason why soccer appeals to so many people is because of its continuous and relatively uninterrupted pace. Great physical demands are placed on a player as they make the transition from offense to defense. Players must be able to sprint intensely for distances of 6 to 60 yards interspersed with slower running or jogging at similar distances. Players are expected to perform these running activities with and without the added skills of stopping, controlling, and accurately passing the ball.

A key component to being a successful player is obtaining the physical fitness level necessary to accomplish these aerobic, anaerobic, and skilled movements. Fitness for soccer must address the areas of flexibility, muscular strength and endurance, and cardiovascular capacity.

This chapter will address each of these areas of fitness and their importance in preventing injuries in soccer. Initially, however, a brief discussion on the ideal pre-participation physical exam will be offered including a physical fitness evaluation.

PRE-PARTICIPATION PHYSICAL EXAMINATION

The athlete's pre-participation examination is an integral part of soccer as well as all athletic programs. This evaluation provides a mechanism by which each athlete is thoroughly screened from a physical stand point as well as from a fitness stand point. It is during this time that any factors restricting or eliminating an individual from participation are identified. However, such physical examinations are affordable only for college soccer players and beyond. Unfortunately, few high school programs provide such extensive examinations. It is advisable that the athletes consult their pediatrician prior to the start of soccer season.

The ideal pre-participation examination is a multi-disciplinary evaluation conducted by a team of specialists ranging from family practitioners and internal medicine physicians to orthopaedic surgeons. Each physician focuses on their area of specialization noting those factors which might restrict or disqualify an individual from safely participating in his/her sport. A history of previous medical problems, a general physical examination including an eye examination, and an orthopaedic examination are the basic areas a pre-season evaluation should include. Factors such as a history of exercise induced asthma, high blood pressure, elevated glucose or protein levels, previous head trauma, single paired organs, torn ligaments or joint pains may warrant further investigation, coaching preparation, or disqualification from participation.

PHYSICAL FITNESS EVALUATION

Endurance: The twelve (12) minute run test is a simple and common way of testing cardiovascular endurance. The test has been proven to correlate well with tests that measure maximum oxygen consumption. A high school and college athlete in excellent condition should be able to cover at least 1.75 miles in twelve minutes For younger athletes, the distance would be adjusted proportionally to the age of the athlete. For example, most 8–9 years olds can run a one mile distance in 7–9 minutes. Girls usually run slightly slower in the upper range of the 7–9 minutes.

Strength: An excellent way of screening an individual for strength is through manual muscle testing techniques. This method, when performed under the observation of a skilled clinician, will point out asymmetries in strength which may warrant further investigation by more sophisticated means, such as isokinetic testing. Another common way to obtain a base line measurement of strength is by using the best score among three (3) trials of a single maximum lift of isotonic weights. It is the authors' opinion that this method should be reserved for those individuals in college or older (if at all) because the risk of injury is high in such activities.

Power: The simplest and most common way of obtaining a base line power measurement is through the vertical jump test. In this test the athlete stands near a wall or measuring device and jumps as high as possible reaching up as they do so. This measurement is compared to the athlete standing and reaching as high as possible without moving or lifting either foot.

Isokinetic devices can also be used to measure power. Testing on such devices, however, is costly and generally impractical unless rehabilitating in a clinical setting.

Flexibility: Three simple tests can be used to assess the flexibility of the lower extremities. The sit and reach test can indicate tightness of the hamstrings or back. For this test, the individual sits on the floor with knees straight and reaches for

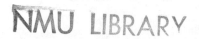

the toes. The sacrum (pelvis) should be perpendicular to the floor. If the individual cannot achieve this position with their pelvis, the hamstrings are too tight. The entire back should form a slow C curve.

To test for flexibility of the calf muscles (plantar flexors), the athlete, sitting with a straight knee, actively dorsiflexes their foot. Using a simple goniometer (measures range of motion) the foot should be able to be pulled back at least 15°. Anything less than this indicates tightness of the calf muscles.

The Thomas test position is an easy and accurate way of assessing the flexibility of the hip flexors, quadriceps, and iliotibial band. The athlete lies supine with the edge of the table hitting him/her about mid-thigh. One knee is pulling up towards the chest, just enough to flatten the lower back against the table, and the other leg is then allowed to relax and drop to the floor. The back of the thigh of the relaxed leg should rest on the table. If not, tightness of the hip flexor is indicated. The knee should rest at a 90° angle. Anything short of this indicates tightness of the quadriceps femoris. Lastly, one should observe if the knee moves away from the mid-line of the body. If so, iliotibial band tightness is indicated.

Proprioception: Proprioception can be defined simply as the body's sensory awareness of its joint and body position in space. Problems with proprioception can arise from injuries such as ankle sprains. Conversely, if the athlete has had a previous injury to a joint and is not completely rehabilitated, poor proprioception can cause an injury. It is therefore wise to perform a simple test to assess the proprioception of each athlete. To evaluate proprioception ask the athlete to simply balance on one foot. Assess their ability to balance on one foot and compare it to their ability to balance on the other foot. To make the test more difficult ask the athlete to close their eyes while balancing on one foot. If the individual has much more difficulty balancing on one foot than the other, further assessment by a health care practitioner (physician, physical therapist, or trainer) and additional rehabilitation may be warranted.

Body composition: Assessing the percentage of body fat a person possesses is important for two reasons. First, it gives the coach, parents, and trainer (if available) the knowledge of how much weight an athlete can loose safely during the season without loosing muscle mass. Well conditioned male athletes normally possess between 8% and 13% body fat while well conditioned female athletes usually possess between 15% and 20%. Secondly, this information can be used to counsel the athlete on the elimination of excessive adipose tissue, leading to a healthier lifestyle and enhanced performance levels.

There are numerous ways of evaluating body fat percentages. Underwater weighing is probably the most accurate way; however, it is often the most impractical. The simplest way of measuring the percentage of body fat is through the use of skin fold calipers. In this method, the tester pinches the subcutaneous fat between the thumb and index finger, pulling it slightly away from the body. The skin fold calipers are used to measure the millimeters of fat present at a particular spot. Generally, six sites are measured on the body. They include the mid-triceps, subscapularis, top of the pelvis, abdominal, upper part of the thigh and mid-axillary regions. Measurements are then plugged into any one of several equations (based on age and sex) which when calculated, provide the evaluator with a percentage of body fat.

PREVENTION THROUGH CONDITIONING

As mentioned earlier, soccer is essentially a running sport wherein the player alternately jogs (aerobic activities) and sprints for relatively short distances (anaerobic activity). Players must also have the explosive power and agility to propel a ball, sprint, jump or change directions quickly.

One of the most effective ways of preventing injuries in any sport is to be in top physical condition before and during the season. Therefore, the remainder of this chapter will address the basic concepts needed to properly design a physical fitness program for soccer players. This discussion will not address the topic of skill training activities. Coaches should be well versed in these skill activities, however.

FLEXIBILITY EXERCISES

Flexibility can be defined as the range of motion available at a specific joint or with any group of muscles. Though often neglected, stretching exercises are familiar to most athletes. A few basic concepts should be kept in mind when developing a flexibility/stretching program.

First, do not stretch cold muscles. Warm up calisthenics or jogging should be performed prior to any stretching program to warm muscles and connective tissue, and thus making them more receptive to being elongated.

The second concept of flexibility to be considered is the technique to employ when stretching tissues. Ballistic stretching consists of using the momentum of the body to bob in an attempt to elongate the muscle. This type of stretching causes certain muscle receptors to be activated which in turns stimulates the activation of muscle fibers. The muscle is thus being stimulated to contract while the individual is attempting to stretch the muscle. Though ballistic stretching has been shown to improve flexibility, this type of stretching has a potential to cause musculoskeletal strains. Ballistic stretching is not recommended for these reasons.

Static stretching consist of slowly stretching muscles to a subpainful threshold and maintaining this position for at least 5 seconds and as long as 20 to 30 seconds. To assure a safe stretch, each stretch should be taken just beyond the point of tightness. Strict form must be adhered to and no movement should be forced.

A thorough stretching program which includes both the upper and lower extremities as well as trunk musculature should be explored prior to practices and game situations.

STRENGTH

Another component of conditioning is strength training. Strength training involves the development of muscular strength, power, and endurance.

To understand strength training one must understand some of the basic physiology of muscle contraction. First, muscles derive their source of energy for muscle contraction from adenosine triphosphate (ATP). ATP, which is synthesized from the food we consume, is utilized in both anaerobic and aerobic energy systems to produce energy (see Chapter 6 for more details).

Aerobic energy systems depend on the availability of oxygen for their production of energy. Carbohydrates, fats, and protein are broken down in the presence of oxygen. This system of energy production allows energy to be supplied to the muscles for several hours.

Another important physiological factor worth noting is that there are two basic types of muscle fibers. Type II fibers (fast twitch fibers) are best adapted for anaerobic types of activities. Conversely, Type I (slow twitch muscle fibers) are better adapted for aerobic or endurance exercises. Both Type I and II muscle fibers can utilize aerobic and anaerobic energy production systems. All muscles are also made up of combinations of both types of fibers. Some individuals have more Type II fibers and are therefore more suited for "power" types of activities such as sprinting and jumping, while other athletes possess more Type I fibers and are therefore adept at endurance types of activities. Training programs must be designed to enhance both the fast and slow twitch fibers since each is needed in soccer (for further details see Chapter 6).

PRINCIPLES IN TRAINING

Building on the foundation of the basic physiological factors, coaches must now consider several principles which must be understood when developing a specific training program for their athletes.

1. **Overload**. The overload principle simply states that in order to build strength, power, endurance or flexibility the activity employed must be such that it exceeds in intensity the demands previously or routinely encountered. The overload principle is the foundation for the progressive principle.

2. **Progressive**. The progressive principle states that as individuals begin applying overloads, improvements (i.e., increased strength and endurance) will be experienced. As this improvement is recognized, progressively greater demands (be

they heavier weights, more wind sprints, longer sprints, etc.) must be imposed or improvement will not be continued.

3. **Specificity**. The principle of specificity is particularly important in soccer. The principle states that training should work the muscle involved in the specific sport in the same manner that they will be utilized during the competition. Furthermore, it encourages the development of the primary energy systems to be utilized during the competitive activity.

A simple example will clarify this principle. It is a fact that soccer involves a great deal of running. If the athlete trains by slowly running 3 to 4 miles per day, they will surely enhance their cardiovascular fitness and their aerobic energy system. Soccer, however, greatly involves the anaerobic energy system. The player must be able to repeatedly run sprints. Therefore, a training/conditioning program which incorporates repeated sprints must be used to improve the strength and muscular endurance necessary to successfully compete in soccer.

4. **Frequency**. Frequency is simply the number of workouts performed in a certain unit of time. To recognize improvement in strength, endurance and skill, training must take place on a regular basis. If players do not regularly train, they will loose the strength, endurance or skill necessary to compete at this demanding sport.

5. **Active Rest**. This is often the most overlooked principle when designing a training program. Muscles do not grow during exercise, they are torn down. Hypertrophy (increased size) of muscles and increased strength of muscles and tendons occurs during the recuperation period. If constantly stressed without adequate rest, muscles and tendons will eventually break down and injuries due to overuse will occur.

Active rest consists of low volume and a low to moderate intensity of work which is designed to allow the tissue to sufficiently recuperate. The activity essentially brings extra blood to the tissue in order to: 1) flush out the waste products (i.e., lactic acid, etc.); 2) bring additional nutrients; and 3) promote healing to the formerly taxed tissue.

A thorough understanding of these five (5) basic principles will allow a skilled coach the ability to design a comprehensive conditioning program for muscle strength and endurance.

CARDIOVASCULAR ENDURANCE

The most essential component of a well conditioned athlete is his/her cardiovascular endurance. Cardiovascular endurance can be defined as the ability of the heart, lungs, and blood vessels to efficiently and effectively carry oxygen to the muscles and their connective tissue while simultaneously removing waste products from these same tissues. Approximately 3 milliliters of oxygen per kilograms per minute is the minimum aerobic requirement everyone possesses. The goal of cardiovascular endurance training (aerobic exercises) is to increase the athletes' maximum aerobic capacity.

Aerobic training affects the human body in several beneficial ways. The stroke volume (amount of blood expelled with each pump of the heart muscle) is increased making the heart a more efficient pump. When the heart rate is increased with exercise the amount of oxygenated blood is significantly increased. In addition, both blood plasma volumes and the amounts of hemoglobin increase with proper training; therefore, the blood can transport more oxygen to the tissues. The receiving tissue also learns how to better utilize the increased oxygen it's being supplied. Blood pressure will be lowered. Furthermore, the body becomes more efficient at removing the waste products from the exercised tissue; thus, fatigue does not set in as quickly (for further details see Chapter 6).

To successfully improve one's cardiovascular fitness the rate of exercise must be intense enough to increase the heart rate to 60% to 80% of its maximal rate. To calculate the maximal heart rate of an individual the following formula is used: 220 minus the age of the person equals maximal heart rate. This intensity must be maintained for 20 to 30 minutes to improve one's aerobic capacity. Furthermore, these workouts (running, bicycling, cross country skiing, swimming etc.) must be performed 3 to 4 times per week. Example: a 15-year-old soccer player would have to achieve a heart rate between 123 and 164 (220 − 15 = 205, 205 × 60% = 123, 205 × 80% = 164), maintained for at least 20 to 30 minutes, 3 times per week, to enhance his/her cardiovascular capacity. There are several ways to achieve this high level of intensity in a soccer practice. Some examples include: having 7 V 7 (or any other combination) with more than 1 ball in order to keep the players marking or chasing the ball; dribbling through cones for 10–15 minute intervals; and scrimmages wherein the soccer ball is quickly provided to the players when it is out of bounds in order to keep the activity continuous.

Chapter

FOUR

Management of Soccer Injuries

Soccer related injures require management both at the time of, and for some time after, the occurrence of an injury. Acute and immediate management is aimed at preventing further damage to tissues until definitive healing and rehabilitation can take place. The removal of the athlete from the field of play immediately following any injury allows the player to rest and gives the coach and the player adequate time to thoroughly evaluate the injury. The key to the immediate management of injuries in most cases is RICE (rest, ice, compression and elevation). RICE is an effective and prudent treatment for most soccer injuries, and involves little if any risk. Injuries that last several days and are associated with pain without remission or with increasing pain should be referred to a physician who has the capability and training necessary to properly evaluate and treat sports related injuries. If an athlete experiences frequent coughing and wheezing after bouts of aerobic activity a consultation with a physician is necessary to determine whether or not the player has exercise-induced asthma; in these cases, there is treatment available which will allow continuation of play.

There are few epidemiological studies that document the type and incidence of soccer injuries in young players and thus there are relatively few generalizations that can be made regarding injuries occurring on a frequent or regular basis. Soccer is appropriately considered a contact sport, which is different from a collision sport, such as American football. In soccer, contact is a part of the game but it occurs as incidental to and not as a planned part of the game. Contact is not used to stop, impede or alter the course of another player, and the upper body is not used to grasp or pull on a regular basis. Thus, in soccer the predominance of injuries occur in the lower extremities (see Figure 4.1).

Direct injuries seen in contact sports are usually due to blunt trauma or a sudden blow to the tissue involved. The severity of the trauma can vary from mild damage to a tissue, to complete rupture of the tissue. The pain associated with these injuries runs the spectrum from mild to severe with varying degrees of functional loss and disability.

WHAT TO DO WHEN AN INJURY OCCURS ON THE FIELD (see Figure 4.2)

Since most youth soccer teams will not have a physician or trainer present, the coach, players, and parents must be prepared to recognize the severity of any injury that occurs during the course of play. If in doubt, the injury must be treated as though it were serious. Fortunately, soccer is a sport that has only a moderate incidence of injury. When an injury does occur, do not immediately move the injured player until you ascertain from your own observations and that of the player the type and severity of the injury. If the player cannot get up on his own, then he should not be moved. The coach should always err on

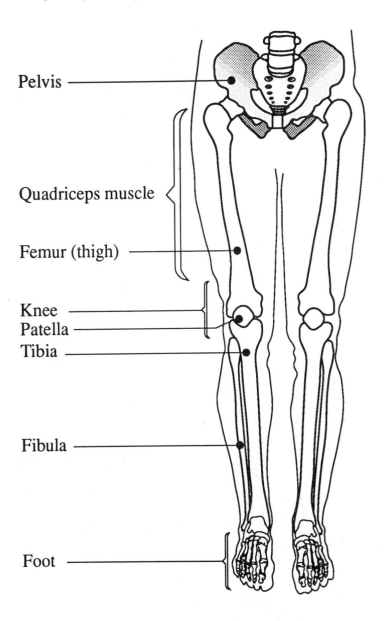

Pelvis

Quadriceps muscle

Femur (thigh)

Knee
Patella
Tibia

Fibula

Foot

Figure 4.1.

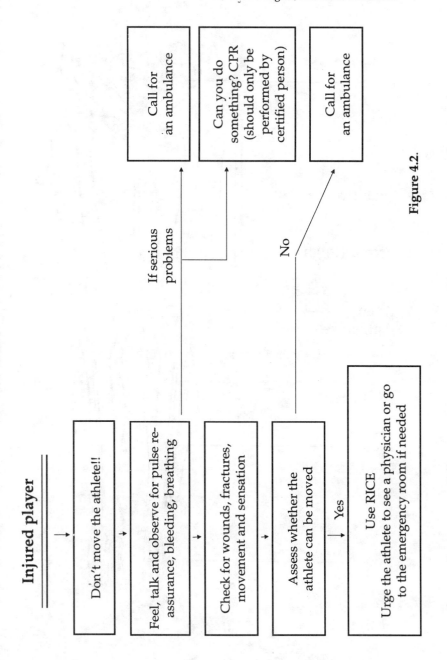

Figure 4.2.

the side of safety. If the player has difficulty with vital signs (breathing, pupil size, pulse, feeling of touch, speech, consciousness), then an ambulance should be called. In extreme situations CPR may have to be given (by a qualified person) if there is severe difficulty in breathing.

Most of these injuries can frequently be treated by simply applying first aid techniques on the field; however, more serious injuries, such as broken bones, require hospital or physician assistance.

Most common injuries in sports are due to overuse. Any physal activity causes changes in the tissue that requires readjustment and a healing period. Overuse of muscles is due to either too much exercise or too frequent exercise within a period of time without a sufficient rest period for recovery. Cross training combining the use of different muscles on different days is valuable in providing rest periods.

If the pattern of overuse continues, it can lead to rupture and damage or failure of the muscle tissues. Common examples of injuries due to overuse include stress fracture and shin splints. The three types of tissue injuries are listed below:

Contusions: This is a blow to soft tissue such as muscles and skin and involves capillary and cellular damage.

Strains: This is an injury to the matrix of a muscle or a tendon (a tendon is the connective tissue which joins the muscle to the bone). This is usually a pulling or traction type injury.

Sprains: This is a partial or complete tear of a ligament. A ligament is a supporting tissue that holds the bones of a joint together and allows motion only in the appropriate plane. A good example is the medial collateral ligament of the knee.

All athletic injuries are caused by either macro-trauma or micro-trauma. Macro-trauma is relatively easy to understand. It occurs when an overload of force is applied to an anatomical structure, and, because the force can not be resisted, the anatomical structure fails mechanically. Micro-trauma occurs subtly. Micro-trauma is caused by repeated small insults and injuries to an anatomical structure. No one small application of force is sufficient to create overload. The small forces occur with enough frequency over a relatively short period of time to compromise a biological mechanical structure. That structure is unable to repair itself rapidly enough to prevent ultimate failure. The most common example of this type of trauma is a stress fracture.

RICE

RICE is an acronym used by trainers and other sports medicine personnel for the initial treatment of most injuries. It stands for rest, ice, compression, and elevation. If there is any question regarding the severity of an injury, this is a reasonable and prudent manner in which to begin treatment.

Rest

Rest may be immediate or delayed, partial or complete. Certainly, in its most basic form rest implies taking an injured player out of the game or practice situation and giving him/her adequate time to recover. In overuse injuries rest may be relative, such as a decreased activity level rather than the complete cessation of activity. Rest for injured body parts may include splints, casts, and non-weight-bearing with crutches.

Ice

Lowering the temperature of a traumatized area to approximately 3 to 4°C Fahrenheit (F) is important to reduce further injury to tissue. This is called cryotherapy. Cryotherapy, an ancient whcih was practiced as far back as the Grecian Empire, involves the use of cooling to reduce trauma to an injured area and to initiate rehabilitation. In any injury, tissue is damaged and the injured region undergoes a healing process. Secondary to the healing process, there are two detrimental occurrences that can cause further tissue damage, and these are enzyme release and hypoxia (reduced oxygen). Hypoxia can cause further cell death which can lead to additional damage. The application of ice to the injured area yields the following benefits:

1. Reduces regional metabolism and oxygen utilization. Cryotherapy results in a greater chance for tissue survival.

2. Reduces degradation of healthy tissue by the enzymes released from the damaged region.

3. Induces vasoconstriction to the damaged area and thus reduces further damage and swelling. Prolonged cryotherapy may allow vasodilation of the area; thus, the intermittent use of ice for 15 to 20 minutes at a time may be more effective than ice alone.

4. Delays inflammation or the actual release of inflammatory enzymes.

5. Has an analgesic affect that often allows proper mobility and prevents a painful reflex arc.

Therefore, the early application of ice after an injury is very helpful in the overall treatment of the injury. Cryotherapy should be applied for 15 to 20 minutes several times a day for the first 48 to 72 hours following an injury. Heat is not recommended in the first two days after an injury. However, after two days contrast treatment, that is alternating heating and cooling, may be used. The use of wet ice is probably the most effective and quickest way to reduce tissue temperature. Wet ice may be more effective than cold packs because it can provide a greater surface area for contact with the injury.

Compression

Compression may be used as a part of splinting or simply to control edema (accumulation of fluids) and swelling. It is important to remember that compression is quite different from strangulation which can cause circulatory compromise. In other words, a modest compression dressing that does not cut off the circulation will help control pain and edema and will help to splint the injured area. The most common method of compression is an elastic wrap, but caution must be exercised not to make the wrap too tight.

Elevation

Elevation is also a method of edema control and helps to ensure rest. Elevation means that the injured body part is elevated in reference to the right side of the heart. The right side of the heart defines the pressure of venous return of the circulatory system or the drainage from an involved limb. Therefore, to effectively elevate a lower extremity, the patient must be in a recumbent position.

It is difficult to decide which injuries are minor and will improve on their own, and which injuries require referral to a consulting physician. Obviously, the extremes are easy to identify as any coach or player can recognize a minor ankle sprain which one can "walk off" and recover from in a matter of minutes. Conversely, a displaced fracture requiring a trip to an emergency room is also easy to identify. The problem arises when there are injuries that effect play on a subtle basis; in these instances, the method of treatment may not be obvious. In these cases the authors recommend referral to an orthopaedic surgeon certified by the American Academy of Orthopaedic Surgeons. One may choose a surgeon who has a special interest and expertise in sports medicine. As a matter of ethics and courtesy, and even financial necessity, depending upon the changes we see in medical practice, it is often appropriate to use a primary care physician to initiate a referral. Many players, both young and old, will more readily consult their coach regarding an injury than parents, family or physician. This may place a burden and responsibility on coaches to attend various coaching seminars on first aid and injury identification.

The remainder of this section will discuss selected injuries that are common to soccer. It is obviously impossible to cover all injuries but an attempt will be made to highlight the injuries that most commonly occur on the soccer field.

LOWER EXTREMITY INJURIES (see Figure 4.1)

1. **Blisters.** The most common injury is the simple blister. In an ideal situation, all soccer players would come to practice with shoes that were well broken in; in addition, the player would have developed appropriate calluses on their feet. Unfortunately, this is not always the case. Frequently, in the beginning of the season players will have new, poorly broken in, or poorly fitted shoes. In addition, often at the beginning of the

season players are not in good physical condition. All of this can lead to blister formation on prominent areas in the foot. A blisters is an irritation of the superficial layer of skin until it looses attachment to the underlying layer; this space is frequently filled with fluid. Blisters should be kept clean. Often an extra pair of socks or adequate padding and a petroleum jelly gauze over a blister will enable the player to continue to participate. The fluid in a blister is generally sterile and routine puncturing of a blister is not advocated. However, at times drainage under sterile conditions or spontaneous drainage or rupture will decompress the blister and allow a more rapid return to play.

2. **Turf Toe**. This is a sprain or injury to the supporting structures around the toe joint from hypertension or repeated hyperextension. In the foot itself, a common injury is a sprain of the 1st metatarsal phalangeal joint, frequently called turf toe (see Figure 4.2). This can occur either from an acute episode, or can be the result of a repetitive injury. It is more frequently seen when playing on a hard surface such as artificial turf or an indoor field. On these surfaces less rigid shoes are used which also contributes to the problem. It is impossible to adequately immobilize this joint for complete healing and still allow continued play; therefore, only rest will cure this injury. Frequently, players with turf toe continue to play; however, the injury will be a nagging problem throughout the season resolving only when the toe is allowed to rest and heal.

3. **Foot**. Twisting injuries to the foot can result in a sprain of the tarsal, metatarsal, or intermetatarsal joints. This can lead to localized swelling, persistent pain, point tenderness and difficulty pushing off the foot. If a player has pain in the mid foot area the foot should be evaluated early with adequate X-rays. If one misses an acute injury and does not treat it until it becomes chronic it may preclude conservative or nonsurgical management. Surgery for a chronically stretched ligament may require arthrodesis which will result in loss of foot motion. A fracture or stress fracture of the navicular may also be present with pain in the mid-foot area (see below).

a. **Flat Foot/Plantar Fasciitis (see Figure 4.3)**. A foot with a relatively flat arch may be predisposed to injury. The most common injury in this situation is plantar fasciitis. This condi-

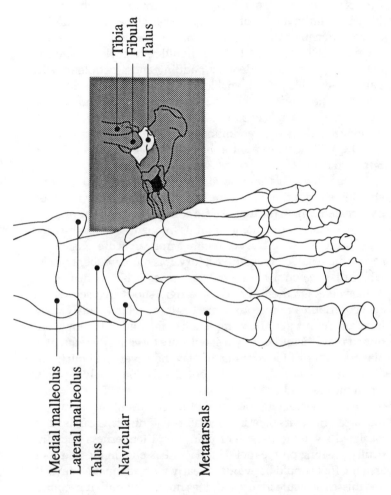

Figure 4.3.

tion results in pain along the plantar fascia which runs along the plantar or under surface of the foot. This tissue acts as a truss to support the normal arch of the foot. If this area is abnormally stretched either acutely or through repetitive loading and unloading of the foot, it may lead to pain which is most often felt at the insertion of the fascia into the heel. The common heel spur is really due to irritation of the plantar fascia as it inserts into the heel itself.

With this type of injury pain along the arch and a stiffness of the foot is felt most acutely upon first arising. The pain decreases a little as the foot is limbered and loosened by walking, but is felt again with increased activity, as the entire complex of symptoms is aggravated by increased activity. Appropriate treatment involves the use of anti-inflammatories, ice, and arch supports or taping. Cases which do not respond to this conservative management scheme need to be referred for expert evaluation to make sure that there is no abnormality in the bony structure of the foot which may play a part in causing this pain.

b. **Sever's Apophysitis**. This is a condition due to relative overuse or micro-trauma seen at the insertion of the Achilles tendon into the heel. There is a growth center or apophysis at the insertion of the tendon that may be aggravated by activity. This area is also prone to inflammation and irritation because of a potential weak point where the tendon inserts near the cartilaginous center of the growth plate. Injuries in this area are best treated symptomatically and should disappear when the player reaches skeletal maturity. Icing, anti-inflammatories and, frequently, a small heel lift will often relieve symptoms. If the heel lift does not provide relief, one can consider prescription orthotics for the treatment of this condition.

c. **Stress Fractures**. Stress fractures are common in the foot. They occur whenever stress or activity induced remodeling of the bone occurs so rapidly that the deossification (the antonym of ossification; ossification is defined as bone formation) stage outstrips the repair stage. This leads to a negative turnover of hard bony tissue. Tenderness and inability to bear weight are the signs and symptoms that contribute to the diagnosis of a stress fracture. Pain that persists, even after cessation of activity, such as in the evening or morning after playing is an important symptom. The most common area of occurrence for stress fractures is the 2nd metatarsal; however, any metatarsal may be affected. Persistent pain in any area in the foot is a mandate for referral and X-ray evaluation. If an X-ray does not show specific changes, a bone scan may be necessary to make the appropriate diagnosis. Almost all stress fractures can be successfully treated with simple restriction of activity. That is, limitation of running, jumping and walking great distances. This type of injury usually does not require splinting or non-weight-bearing treatment. Treated in this manner stress fractures almost always heal, but if a stress fracture is ignored it is not inconceivable that the patient may go on to fracture through the stress fracture converting it to a displaced fracture that needs more aggressive treatment. There are several stress fractures which require greater vigilance and more aggressive treatment. One of these is a stress fracture at the base of the 5th metatarsal. A stress fracture in this area must be watched carefully as these have a potential for nonunion and can require operative intervention. Another area of concern is the navicular. This is the bone in the mid-foot area where the 1st and 2nd metatarsals join the mid-foot. Fractures of this bone are best treated with non-weight-bearing and immobilization. Unrecognized fractures of the navicular may lead to arthritis, and can require a fusion for successful treatment. While this may decrease pain, it will significantly limit motion in the foot. If there is reproducible point tenderness to palpation in any bone in the foot, one must consider referral for evaluation of a stress fracture.

d. **Sprain (see Figure 4.4).** A sprain is a medical term which describes a torn ligament. The most common ankle injury seen in all sports, including soccer, is the lateral ankle sprain. The ankle is a mortise and tenon joint with inherent bony stability. The lateral ligaments are the weaker ligaments in this joint compared to the medial ligaments. There are three lateral ligaments that attach the fibula, or outside bone of the leg, to the talus and calcaneus of the foot. These ligaments prevent the ankle from rolling over or inverting. A sprain to these ligaments occurs when a player lands on the outside of his foot in such a manner as to twist his body over it or roll the foot underneath. The degree of the tear can vary. Significant tears which do not cause limping can be successfully treated with icing and strap-

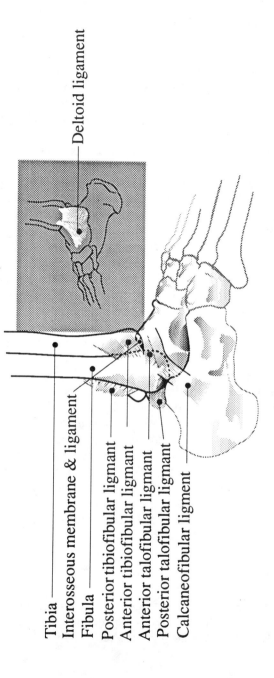

Deltoid ligament

Tibia
Interosseous membrane & ligament
Fibula
Posterior tibiofibular ligmant
Anterior tibiofibular ligmant
Anterior talofibular ligmant
Posterior talofibular ligmant
Calcaneofibular ligment

Figure 4.4.

ping, and one might continue play while a minor sprain heals. More significant sprains will need support of the ankle through taping, strapping, or braces, and some of these treatments will allow resumption of play in orthotic devices. Significant sprains require X-ray evaluation because there is no other way to insure that one does not have a fracture. It is important to remember that younger players have an epiphysis (growth plate) at the tip of the fibula which is just as likely to be injured as the ligament. In fact, it is relatively common for the epiphysis to be injured or even avulsed or pulled off because the junction of the epiphysis to the bone itself is weaker than the ligament. If the epiphyseal injury is nondisplaced, this can be treated with immobilization just as with a severe sprain, but the injury should be recognized and properly diagnosed. The degree of swelling and the degree of functional impairment are the determining factors in deciding whether or not to refer the player to a physician for evaluation. Treatment may require a period of immobilization in order to allow the sprain to heal; once the sprain has healed, protective devices such as splints or braces and taping should be utilized in order to allow an early return to play. It is important to make sure that normal mobility and strength is restored to the ankle prior to full return to unrestricted activity. A referral to a certified trainer or physical therapist may expedite rehabilitation.

Medial ankle sprains or deltoid ligament sprains are rarer than those just discussed above, and can be treated in a similar manner. Again, in cases of persistent swelling and soreness it is important to get an X-ray to avoid missing a fracture, particularly of a growth center. The mechanism that causes a sprain can also cause an avulsion fracture off the base of the 5th metatarsal. This is a smaller piece of bone and more proximal than the stress related fracture. These fractures will most often heal with minimal rest and immobilization.

LEG

Clearly, the most common injuries to the leg are contusions and hematomas from contact, either with another player or another player's foot. Appropriate shin guards prevent many of these injuries, but it would be rare for a soccer player to go through an entire season without sustaining a contusion to the leg. It is important to treat these injuries with extra pads; in particular, a foam doughnut can be made in order to protect or take pressure off a sore area. Shin guards can be placed over this.

a. **Compartment Syndrome.** The muscles in the lower extremity of the leg, particularly those in the anterior compartment, are invested with a thick supporting tissue called fascia. This forms a rigid sleeve around the muscle and a contusion, fracture, or even extreme overuse can cause the muscle to swell inside of this confining tissue. Swelling can create pressure to such a degree that it can cut off the relatively low pressure capillary inflow which the muscle depends upon for its nourishment. Compartment syndrome occurs when the pressure leads to ischemia or a loss of blood supply to the muscle. This type of injury constitutes a surgical emergency and requires release of this tight structure in order to allow the muscle to survive. The hallmark of this diagnosis is severe pain in the muscle itself. Lack of a pulse distal to the involved area has also been described as a part of this syndrome, but frequently a pulse may be readily apparent while the muscle above is still ischemic. Paresthesias, "funny feelings," or numbness are common, but anyone with severe pain should be evaluated on an emergency basis, because the only reliable way to exclude acute compartment syndrome is with direct measurements of the tissue pressure.

b. **Stress Fracture.** A very common area for stress fractures is the tibia. It is often difficult to differentiate a stress fracture from shin splints; however, stress fractures seem to have a more focused or localized area of direct tenderness to palpation and require a period of rest. The diagnosis is usually made by X-rays, but occasionally the X-rays are normal. If several X-rays are normal and pain is persistent, it is worthwhile to obtain a bone scan to make sure that there is not a stress fracture that is not yet apparent. Again, the treatment for stress fractures is avoidance of impact activity. This type of injury does not prevent one from bearing weight, but running should be prohibited. Consequently, sports activities may be prohibited until the fracture is healed, usually over a 6 to 8 week period. It is important to remember, however, that non-weight-bearing activities and fitness activities such as biking and swimming can be used to maintain fitness during the healing period. Weight training may be included in the rehabilitation and is not contraindicated by stress fractures.

c. **Shin Splints**. Shin splints are most frequently caused by overtraining. They are probably best described as a reactive peritendinitis or an inflammation of the insertion of a muscle into the bone. There are some anatomic conditions which predispose players to the development of shin splints; in these cases, the incidence of shin splints can be decreased with appropriate foot wear and orthotics. However, the essential factor in the prevention of shin splints is a gradual increase in training coupled with adequate flexibility. Sometimes it is extremely difficult to differentiate between shin splints and a stress fracture without an X-ray or a bone scan. The severity and frequency of the pain leads one to make a clinical judgement as to the appropriate time for obtaining these studies.

There are, as mentioned, certain conditions that have a causal effect with regard to shin splints. One condition is overtraining and another is an anatomic predisposition. When players stay fit in a year round conditioning program overtraining is less of a problem. An athlete should gradually, but not precipitously increase the amount of running. Predisposition of an anatomic nature usually involves mechanical problems with the lower foot. This can include an extremely rigid and highly arched foot or a very flexible flat foot. Either of these conditions prevents the proper damping of forces throughout the lower extremity when the foot and lower limb are exposed to the constant pounding and impact seen with running. Properly fitted orthotics or shoe inserts are often very helpful in this situation, particularly when coupled with the appropriate use of modalities such as ice.

KNEE (see Figure 4.5)

The knee is frequently injured in many sports and is often a source of pain and disability. When dealing with young athletes it is important to remember that hip pain may be referred to in

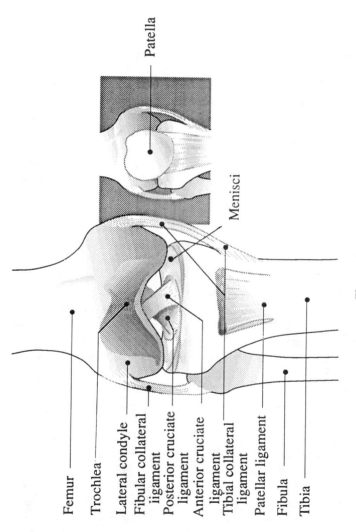

Patella

Menisci

Femur
Trochlea
Lateral condyle
Fibular collateral
ligament
Posterior cruciate
ligament
Anterior cruciate
ligament
Tibial collateral
ligament
Patellar ligament
Fibula
Tibia

Figure 4.5.

the knee much in the way that someone suffering from a heart attack feels pain radiating down his arm. If a young player is complaining of knee pain particularly with a lack of localized findings about the knee, consideration should be given to evaluation of the player's hip as well. When dealing with the knee, it is helpful to think of general categories of injuries and problems. The first would be knee stability, the second the extensor mechanism and its various afflictions, and the third would be internal derangements of the knee. Internal derangement are problems that exclude the extensor mechanism or stability but can cause significant knee malfunction.

a. **Stability**. The knee as a joint operates within certain degrees of freedom. It is allowed to bend and extend in some planes but is restricted in others. It is allowed to rotate in a limited manner but is tethered by the ligaments to prevent it from excess motion in certain directions. The ligaments are composed of thickened connective tissue and are attached to either side of the knee joint. The most commonly injured ligament is the medial collateral ligament which is a broad flat ligament that runs down from the medial femoral condyle to the tibia. Thus, it runs down the inside of the knee and crosses the joint acting like a leather strap or hinge. This ligament allows the knee to bend and extend but stops the lower leg from moving away from the body or to the side. The most common injury is when someone is struck from the outer aspect of the knee and the knee bends inward. This stretches or damages the medial collateral ligament. Most of these injuries or sprains require a period of immobilization to allow a damaged ligament to heal. Milder injuries may be treated with mobility and a hinged brace. In younger players there are growth centers or epiphyses about the knee that may be weaker than the ligament. Unlike a ligament injury, in young players, the growth center may be pulled apart or opened up; thus, a subtle widening of this epiphysis may be seen on X-ray. This indicates a fracture through the growth center rather than a ligamentous injury. In other cases ligaments may pull off or avulse a small piece of bone. All significant injuries to the knee should be evaluated with an X-ray.

The next common ligament injury of importance involves the tear of the anterior cruciate ligament. The anterior cruciate is a ligament that is inside the knee, and it runs from the tibia, or lower bone, of the knee to the femur, or upper bone. It runs obliquely across the center of the knee from the anterior medial or inside portion of the tibia to the posterior superior and lateral or outside aspect of the femur. This ligament is injured with twisting or with a sudden deceleration or stop on the knee accompanied with a twist. It can also be injured by a severe force applied to the outer aspect of the knee which first damages the medial collateral; when this ligament is completely torn, anterior cruciate ligament may also be damaged. An injury to this ligament results in significant knee swelling with disability whenever the player or patient attempts to change directions quickly. In most patients damage to this ligament will prevent successful participation in soccer because a soccer player must obviously be able to plant and push off either leg and kick with the other. Injuries to this major ligament to the knee must be referred to the appropriately trained person for treatment, as this ligament can not be repaired without surgery.

b. **Extensor Mechanism**. The extensor mechanism consists of the quadriceps muscles, or the anterior thigh muscles, with their tendon inserting into the patella. The patella, or kneecap, and the patellar tendon, which is the tendon beneath the kneecap, joins this mechanism to the tibia. Thus, when the quadriceps muscles contract they extend or straighten the knee. This is the strong muscle of the anterior thigh that propels the body forward when the leg is planted on the ground. Injuries to the muscles themselves will be discussed below under thigh injuries. The kneecap may be damaged in many ways; for example, a direct blow may cause a contusion.

Sometimes the kneecap will slip or be forced off to the side of the knee thus dislocating or subluxating it from its position. Subluxation is a partial dislocation of the kneecap which is quickly pulled back into place. Milder forms of subluxation that occur over time may be treated effectively with an exercise program and perhaps knee alignment braces. These braces are made of soft neoprene or rubber with a hole cut out for the kneecap and a pad on the side to prevent the kneecap from sliding laterally. These braces are quite light and do not preclude player participation at a high level. The more severe forms of this condition will become evident and may require surgical treatment. This type of knee injury surgery should not be entertained as a solution until a course of nonoperative management has been attempted and found to fail. One exception is an acute injury with a one time forceful dislocation of the kneecap. This is a true traumatic event and may necessitate immediate repair. Fractures of the kneecap may require surgery, but this depends on the nature of the fracture seen on the X-ray.

c. **Tendon**. Below the kneecap is the patellar ligament (or tendon). This tendon attaches the kneecap to the tibia. This is the last link through which the force is transmitted from the muscle to the lower leg. This tendon is often stressed by repetitive use and pounding on the leg as seen in running sports, particularly on hard surfaces. Frequently, tendinitis may occur from relative overuse. Counter force braces or padding, ice, and, again, a gradual increase in the level of activity are the best ways to prevent and treat these types of injury.

Osgood Schlatter's disease is a special type of irritation of the patellar tendon. This occurs in an athlete with an open epiphysis or growth center in the knee. The patellar tendon attaches directly to this area and so this area is a potentially weak spot. Repeated stress on the patella tendon may cause injury and fragmentation to the growth center. This condition is usually reversible and is treated with a counter force brace, with limited running but continuation of play.

d. **Internal Derangement**. The term internal derangement of the knee encompasses many different areas. The three most common areas include plica syndrome, meniscal tears and, particularly in adolescence, osteochondritis dissecans.

(1) **Plica Syndrome**. A plica is a fold of synovial tissue that stretches across the inside of the knee. It is often a normal finding but can become symptomatic if this tissue becomes inflamed, scarred and hardened. When this occurs the tissue can rub or irritate the knee when the knee goes through a

course of flexion and extension. It may result in pain and swelling in the knee. Symptoms include frequent pain on the inside aspect of the knee over the femur; at times, the plica can actually be felt through the skin. Conservative or early treatment consists of the proper use of ice and anti-inflammatories, and can even include a course of supervised physical therapy. When this pain becomes intractable to the point that it interferes with activity and can not be controlled by conservative management, arthroscopy and excision of the plica by surgical methods may be indicated.

(2) **Meniscus**. The meniscus is a fibrocartilaginous tissue that can act as a washer or spacer and shock absorber inside the knee. There are two of these structures in each knee forming an inter and outer or medial and lateral meniscus. They are semicircular in shape and embrace the condyles of the femur. The meniscus is attached to the joint and can be damaged in twisting type injuries. If a meniscus is completely torn, surgical excision or repair may be required. The signs of a meniscal injury include recurrent swelling of the knee, pain, and tenderness, particularly along the joint line. At times, prior to considering arthroscopic or surgical intervention, special imaging procedures such as MRI (Magnetic Resonance Imaging) may be helpful in making the diagnosis. MRI is an expensive test, and should be used only when necessary; at times, it is more appropriate to proceed to arthroscopic evaluation without an MRI.

(3) **Osteochondritis Dissecans**. Largely seen in adolescence, this condition occurs when a portion of the joints' surface, or more precisely, the bone directly under the cartilage surface of the joint may temporarily loose its blood supply. This can result in fragmentation of the cartilaginous surface of the bone. Often, resting the knee or cast immobilization will allow this injury to heal. Occasionally, operative treatment is required, particularly if there are free fragments in the knee. The signs of this injury are swelling and pain. There is often tenderness to direct palpation or touch, particularly when the knee is flexed by the examiner. This diagnosis can frequently be made with plain X-

rays, but at times MRI may be required to confirm the diagnosis.

In summary, the warning signs for significant knee injuries are pain, swelling, locking, or instability. These are injuries that should be fully evaluated prior to resumption of play in order to prevent further injury.

THIGH

Strains and contusions of the thigh muscles are the main injuries occurring in the thigh. Strain implies a tearing of the muscle fibers when a sudden acute overload is applied to them. This is most commonly seen in the quadriceps muscle. The quadriceps are the muscles that extend the knee; when someone is sprinting, they may overload the muscle and tear the fibers. This, as with most muscle injuries, should be treated with rest in order to facilitate healing. These injuries almost never require surgery and can be treated in a conservative manner. A major mistake which is often made is an early return to play based on the fact that the player feels better, but the muscle, while having partially healed, has not healed well enough to allow vigorous activity. An early return to activity can result in frequent reinjuries and prolonged disability. As with any other injury acute injuries are treated with ice.

The adductor muscles are also commonly injured in this manner. This is frequently referred to as a groin pull or strain. The muscles that are tender or damaged are the ones that pull the leg into the mid-line or adduct. Appropriate stretching and warm-up will prevent a lot of these injuries from occurring or recurring. In the acute instance, a certain amount of rest is required. Taping and strapping has been found to be helpful in symptomatic relief, but one must be mindful of the fact that this is a physiological injury, and must be given time to heal.

Often in a younger patient an injury to the entire quadriceps mechanism will result in an avulsion of bone from the pelvis. This can occur because the muscle inserts into a relatively weak area on the bone and the muscle contraction and muscle tensile strength is stronger than that of its insertion into the bone. A similar injury can occur with the hamstring muscles as well. Thus, if there is any severe pain or swelling, particularly at the bony insertion of the muscle, an X-ray of the pelvis may be helpful in making a diagnosis. These bony avulsions seldom require surgery or reattachment, but do indicate the severity of the injury and are helpful in determining the amount of rest necessary.

Contusions of the thigh muscles are seen when a hard object such as a foot or a ball or even another player's head strikes the anterior thigh area. This results in the well known "charlie horse." Obviously, these are difficult to prevent as they are a common mishap which occurs during a play. Once these injuries do occur it is critical to ice them immediately to prevent bleeding and residual stiffness and soreness. Compressive wraps, non-weight-bearing and rest until the muscle can be stretched out and function in a normal contractual manner again are the major treatments for this injury.

HIP

The most common injuries to the hip are mentioned above (that is, bony injuries), but there is another form of bony injury that is also quite painful. This is the "hip pointer." This type of injury refers to an avulsion or an injury through a contusion to the abdominal muscles off the superior edge of the pelvis or hip. This can be quite painful and difficult to control and may require rest for a period of time. Ice and anti-inflammatories as well as rest are the appropriate treatments for this type of injury.

One potentially disastrous problem seen in the hip is the slipped capital femoral epiphysis. In a growing child with open epiphyses even the simple forces of daily activity can cause the growth center of the end of the femur or the round head that inserts in the hip socket to slip. This is truly an emergency situation in that neglect or improper early care can lead to severe arthritic changes in the hip which are difficult to salvage by any means. Thus, if a patient has any limping or loss of motion around the hip, it is important to realize that this particular condition can occur with very little trauma.

UPPER EXTREMITY INJURIES

Upper extremity injuries occur much less commonly during soccer than injuries to the lower extremity, but none the less they can occur. They are usually caused by a fall or associated with a collision.

1. **Shoulder.** In the shoulder the most common injury seen in soccer is an acromioclavicular joint separation or a shoulder separation. Shoulder pads are never worn in soccer, nor should this occasional injury imply that they should be worn. When a player lands directly on the point of the shoulder, the acromioclavicular joint can be disrupted causing a separation or sprain of that joint. The player will experience tenderness directly over the AC joint and may even have the arm sag or the end of the clavicle ride up if the joint is completely disrupted. The degree of the sprain can be confirmed or more fully diagnosed with the appropriate use of X-rays. It is rare that these injuries require surgery in a soccer player, however, a severe injury (called Grade III in medical jargon) with bone tenting the skin may best be treated with surgery. Making the decision as to whether or not to operate will require consultation with a specialist and appropriate X-ray evaluation. The majority of these injuries, are mild and, if there is no obvious deformity, they can be treated with ice and a gradual resumption of play. At times, it is difficult for the player to initially raise his arm over his head and that particular player may not be able to throw the ball into play until his shoulder heals.

2. **Hand and Wrist Injuries.** Hand and wrist injuries are most commonly seen in the goal tender but they can occur in any player who falls. A ball striking the end of the finger can disrupt the extensor mechanism and this can result in a drop finger or mallet finger. When this type of injury occurs, the player is unable to actively extend the DIP or tip joint of the finger;

however, the finger itself can be passively extended. Mallet finger is treated with a splint holding the finger in extension for at least 6 weeks; in addition, an X-ray should be taken to make sure that there is no significant fracture which could require surgical intervention. The decision to play with a splint immobilizing the finger and increasing risk for further injury must be made under advisement and after discussion with the patient, and when appropriate, his or her parents. Various other injuries may occur to the joints, ligamentous sprains, muscle strains, etc. The cardinal rule is that if there is significant swelling in any joint or loss of motion that does not resolve itself within several days, it is wise to refer that individual for appropriate evaluation and X-rays as untreated fractures and sprains can result in irreversible damage to the fine joints of the hand. Many times appropriate splinting will allow a patient to play even with an injury. Sometimes, even though these splints are very small, officials may find them illegal, and it has been the practice of many trainers and coaches to hide the splint under layers of tape thereby making it a legal device.

3. **1st MP or Thumb**. A common injury in all sports is the so-called Gamekeeper's thumb. This term describes a sprain of the ulnar collateral ligament of the MP joint of the thumb where the thumb joins the hand. This injury is due to a subacute stretching of the ligament; during athletic activity, a fall or a collision of the thumb with somebody else can cause the thumb to be driven away from the hand, resulting in this type of injury. There is tenderness and swelling at the metacarpal phalangeal joint. If there is major instability it usually requires surgical repair. If it is minor it can be treated with appropriate splinting and strapping.

4. **Head and Neck**. Injuries to the head and neck may occur in any sport. If a player loses consciousness it is the authors' belief that the patient should be removed from play and not allowed to resume play until evaluated by a physician over a course of several days. If a player suffers from dizziness, nausea or has difficulty with memory, it is imperative that the patient be transported immediately for medical evaluation. With regard to head injuries, it is important to remember that

any injury caused by a force severe enough to cause unconsciousness has the capability of causing a neck injury at the same time. Thus, when someone suffers a severe head injury it is prudent to immobilize the neck until that player can be evaluated properly. Any severe injury to the neck itself should be treated with appropriate immobilization. If there is any significant sensory loss, that is loss of feeling anywhere, that player must be immobilized on the field prior to any transportation. If there are not trained personnel available, the best course of action is not to move the player until such time that emergency medical personnel arrive. This is a severe injury and can be made worse by ill-considered early motion of the patient. The neck should be stabilized and the patient's airway maintained as best as possible until trained help is available.

EXERCISE INDUCED ASTHMA (EIA)

About one in ten persons have asthma. In most cases, asthma is exhibited within the first 15 minutes of exercise. It is also referred to as exercise-induced bronchospasm (EIB). The term bronchospasm refers to the constriction of the air passages in the tracheobronchial tree. EIB is also exacerbated during exercise in cold weather. The most relevant symptoms include breathlessness, coughing, and wheezing. At the onset of such symptoms, the athlete should be removed from playing, rested, and the player's anxiety lowered. At a later time, if the coach, the athlete, or parent is confronted with these symptoms after a short interval of exercise, the athlete should consult a physician to check for asthma. In no way should asthma prevent a player from enjoying soccer. There are several therapeutic measures the physician usually prescribes. Among them — a prolonged warm-up time in order to reduce bronchoconstriction. The physician may prescribe inhalers with a short or long-term bronchodilation effect. Some inhalers can be used within 15 minutes before exercise and/or days before exercise. One of the authors (AES) has an under 15-year-old girls soccer team with nine out of sixteen players on asthma inhaler medication.

FURTHER GENERAL READING

Knight, K.L. (1985) *Cryotherapy Theory, Technique and Physiology*. Chattanooga Corporation, Chattanooga, Tennessee.

Kellett, J. (1986). Acute Soft Tissue Injuries — A Review of the Literature, *Med. Sci. in Sports Exerc.* 18:489–500.

Landry, G.L., and Gomez, J.E. (1991). Management of Soft Tissue Injuries. *Adol. Med. State of the Art Revs.* 2:125–140.

Bocobo C. et al. (1991). The Effect of Ice on Intra-articular Temperature in the Knee of the Dog, *Am. J. of Phys. and Med. Rehab.* 70:181–185.

Belitsky, R.B., et al. (1987). Evaluation of the Effectiveness of Wet Ice, Dry Ice, and Cryogenic Packs in Reducing Skin Temperature, *Phys. Therapy*, 67:1080–1084.

Clarkson, P.M., et al. (1992). Muscle Function After Exercise-Induced Muscle Damage and Rapid Adaptation, *Med. and Sci. in Sports and Exerc.* 24:512–520.

Mahler, Donald A. (1993). Exercise-Induced Asthma, *Med. Sci. Sports Exerc.*, 25:554–561.

Chapter

FIVE

Water and Electrolyte Balance for Soccer Players

Water is the most important nutrient for the soccer player before, during and after the game. During exercise, all of the energy expenditure leads to a large amount of heat production. Evaporation of water through the skin (i.e., sweating) is the critical avenue for cooling and maintaining the core body temperature. The evaporated water which is lost should be replenished in order to restore the normal blood and cellular ionic concentrations which are vital to normal functions. In addition, drinking cold water can cool the body and maintain it at 37°C. The player should drink 1–2 glasses of cold water prior to the practice/game. Also, the player should drink 1 glass of water for every 1 lb weight loss during a practice/game. During the practice/game, the player should drink 4–6 ounces of water every 15–20 minutes to insure proper hydration and well being. If the body temperature is not maintained at 37°C, the following heat-related illnesses (in order of increasing seriousness) can occur: heat cramps; heat exhaustion; and heat stroke.

Water is the most critical nutrient for the survival and well being of a person. One can survive without the intake of other nutrients for days, weeks, and even months but one cannot survive without water for more than a few days. In a 70 Kg (154 lb) person, the water content is about 40 liters (10.56 gallons) (i.e., 60% of body weight). Most of the water (25 liters) is inside cells; nevertheless, about 15 liters reside outside of cells. The blood volume is about 5 liters (1.32 gallons) and the main-tenance of this volume is critical to a person's survival, despite the fact that daily fluid intake can vary from 1–8 liters. Excess fluid intake can easily be regulated; however, a problem arises when fluid intake is below one liter per day and blood volume starts to decrease below 5 liters (for example, a blood volume of 4 liters or less can cause death). Under sedentary conditions the skin and the kidneys (i.e., urine output) are the most important regulators of body water. Under conditions of hot weather and exercise (despite fluid intake in many cases), the skin (because of sweating) becomes the only important regulator of body water, as well as body temperature. Loss of water in a heavy, prolonged exercise (e.g., a 3-hour marathon) can increase from 0.1 to 5 liters.

Sweating is an absolute necessity in maintaining constant body temperature. The sweat rate usually corresponds to in-creases in energy expenditure by the athlete. Trained athletes have more sensitive sweating systems than non-athletes due to adaptation to repetitive exercise. For example, a marathon runner's fluid losses (despite fluid intake in many cases) can consist of 12% of body water and 8% of body weight. Greater than 2% weight loss secondary to water loss from exercise induces severe demands on the thermoregulatory and cardio-vascular systems. Fluid losses during adult soccer games have been reported to be 1 to 3% of body weight. In hot weather, fluid losses can climb to 5% of body weight. Obviously, such a loss should be dealt with in a serious manner.

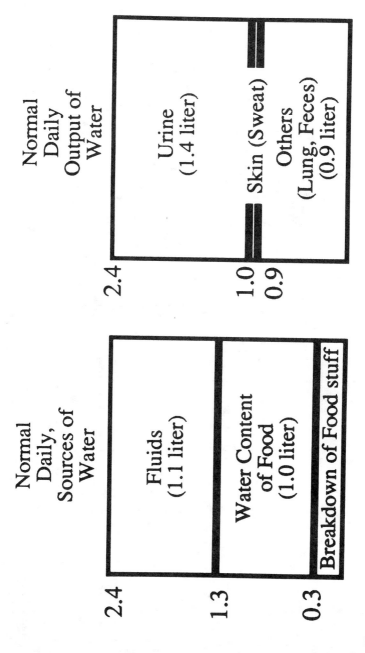

Figure 5.1. An example of the daily amount of water intake (first bar) and output (second bar) for a sedentary person. The numbers given are approximate guesses for normal environmental conditions of temperature and humidity.

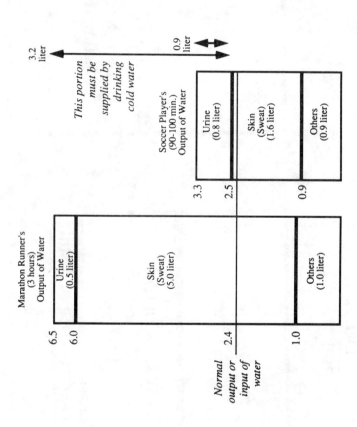

Figure 5.2. An example of the daily required amounts of water needed to be consumed by a marathon runner (3 hours) and a soccer player (90–100 minutes). The values given are approximate for normal environmental conditions of temperature and humidity.

All of the energy expenditure during exercise results in heat. Therefore, body temperature will rise rapidly during exercise if cooling due to sweating does not occur. The prolonged increase in body temperature will eventually cause serious damage to the thermoregulatory system, which can result in serious damage to the body's most sensitive organ — the brain. Thirst, unfortunately, is not a reliable indicator of water loss or rise in body temperature during exercise (or under any stressful condition, particularly in young athletes). Therefore, athletes should drink water not just to quench their thirst, but as part of their exercise regime. Figures 5.1 and 5.2 represent a hypothetical daily water output and water intake for people who are sedentary, who have run a 3 hour marathon, or are playing soccer (90–100 minutes). The numbers are rough estimates, and are only for illustrative purposes. The most scientific way to determine optimal water intake is to weigh the player before and during the game. The loss of weight due to water loss should be adjusted by drinking the same amount of water. Remember, it is better to drink more than less water. The athlete should drink 1–2 glasses of water before the practice/game and 1 glass of water for every 1 lb weight loss during the event. Alternatively, the athlete could do well by simply drinking 4–6 ounces of water every 15–20 minutes during the event. The water should be cold for two reasons; cold water provides a greater capacity to lower core body temperature and it quickens the emptying of the stomach content into the intestines where water absorption occurs.

Children utilize more metabolic energy than adults in performing the same task, and thus they produce more heat. Fortunately, children dissipate heat more efficiently than adults due to a larger surface area to mass ratio. However, when the ambient temperature is hot and humid, the dissipation of heat is inhibited and thus children may be at a greater risk of heat related illnesses than adults during exercise.

Electrolytes such as Na^+, K^+, Cl^-, Ca^{2+} and Mg^{2+} are very important ions and their concentrations in the cell and blood are critical for maintaining normal body function. As we sweat more during exercise, the amount of these ions in the sweat is less than that of the blood. In other words, the body is losing more water than ions. Under heavy exercise conditions, the body loses about 5–7 grams of sodium chloride. However, there is a minimal loss of K^+ and Mg^{2+}. Under conditions of continued exercise (up to 80–90 minutes) there is a need to replenish water continuously, but not salt. If there is heavy exercise beyond the 80–90 minutes, salt replenishment is appropriate. The use of salt tablets during the early phase of exercise (as in most cases of soccer) is detrimental to the body. The body fluid has a higher salt concentration after exercise than before; therefore, the body needs pure water to bring the blood composition back to normal levels. The presence of ions in drinking water does slightly facilitate water absorption through the intestines and its retention in the body. It is because of this fact that "sport drinks" advocates (primarily companies that sell them) promote drinking "sport drinks" for rehydration. However, since the health risks from dehydration far outweighs the risks taken because of a small amount of salt depletion (not present in most youth soccer players due to the limited amount of true activity), it is therefore of paramount importance to first ensure proper hydration with water. However, if the player has two games per day (such as in tournaments), it is then advisable to drink juices or "sports drinks" which contain salt, particularly after each match. After practice/game, the soccer player should ingest large amounts of carbohydrates in order to replenish muscle glycogen content. The ingestion of carbohydrates within the first two hours after play is preferred because it is at this time that muscles have an enhanced capacity to synthesize glycogen.

HEAT RELATED ILLNESSES

Heat Cramps

Heat cramps are similar to other muscle cramps, and may be due to sudden blows, over exercise, lack of blood supply, etc.

Cause: Reduced blood flow to the muscle due to: loss of water, prolonged loss of minerals, etc.

Symptoms: Spasmodic tonic contraction of a given muscle (e.g., abdominal and extremities).

Onset: Gradual or sudden.

Danger: None if treated. Heat cramps could lead to termination of that particular exercise for a few days.

Prevention: Proper physical fitness, proper warm-ups and stretching exercises prior to the activity, and proper hydration.

Treatment: Termination of activity, drinking water, stretching, rest and ice treatment necessary.

Heat Exhaustion

Cause: Loss of water.

Symptoms: Tiredness, weakness, malaise, and feeling progressively weaker, anxiety, dizziness, at times fainting, and hot/dry skin. Persons will experience sweating, a small urine volume, and perhaps unconsciousness.

Onset: Gradual; over several days.

Danger: Rarely, the player may go into shock because of reduced blood volume. However, typically heat exhaustion is not an emergency condition. If not treated, this illness can lead to heat stroke.

Prevention: Proper physical fitness and proper hydration before and during exercise.

Treatment: Termination of activity, rest in a recumbent position, cooling down, drinking water, and later drinking large amounts of mineral rich fluid such as diluted (1:3) fruit and vegetable juices.

Heat Stroke

Brain cells in the hypothalamus maintain body temperature close to 37°C (98.6 °F). These cells respond to the temperature of the blood that passes through them. The cells regulate body temperature by sending signals to release skin vasodilators in order to increase sweating. When rectal temperatures reach 41–43°C, unconsciousness may occur; if that happens, the mortality rate ranges from 50–70%. Heat stroke is the second biggest cause of death after accidental death among athletes.

Cause: Loss of water and a sudden uncontrolled rise in body temperature due to the failure of the thermoregulatory center in the brain.

Symptoms: Heat stroke should be treated as a life threatening *Medical Emergency* as it may lead to death or irreversible damage. The person shows behavioral or mental status changes during heat stress. Symptoms include: a sense of impending doom, headache, dizziness, confusion hysteria and weakness. The person exhibits hot and dry skin, rapid pulse and low blood pressure. Factors which could lead to heat stroke include:

a.   environmental high temperature and high humidity.

b.   high rectal temperature.

c.   hot dry skin (i.e., sweating stops).

d.   cardiorespiratory (e.g., rapid weak pulse, low blood pressure) and central nervous system disturbances.

e.   clouded consciousness and finally, collapse.

Onset: Sudden.

Danger: Brain damage and death is imminent if not treated quickly.

Prevention: Proper physical fitness and proper hydration before and during the exercise.

Treatment:

1.   Call for an ambulance.

2.   Remove clothes and cool in anyway possible with ice and cold water on the body.

3.   Monitor vital signs. (i.e., breathing, heart beat, pupil size).

4.   Massage extremities to promote cooling.

5.   Once the body temperature cools and the person is quite alert, remove from cold environment to prevent hypothermia.

6.   Do not attempt to force water on an unconscious individual as they will choke on it.

Heat Illness Chart

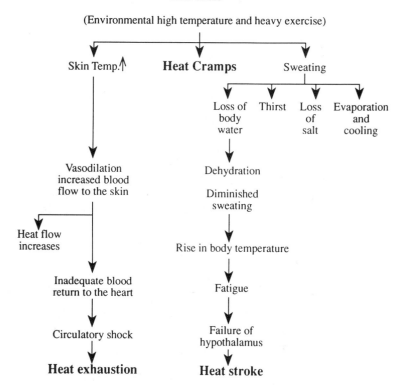

Heat Stress

(Environmental high temperature and heavy exercise)

Skin Temp.↑ | **Heat Cramps** | Sweating

Loss of body water | Thirst | Loss of salt | Evaporation and cooling

Vasodilation increased blood flow to the skin

Dehydration

Diminished sweating

Heat flow increases

Inadequate blood return to the heart

Rise in body temperature

Fatigue

Circulatory shock

Failure of hypothalamus

Heat exhaustion

Heat stroke

Figure 5.3. Flowchart of heat related illnesses and the relevant pathways that lead to heat cramps, heat exhaustion, and heat stroke.

In the hospital, the personnel may perform the following:

1. Administer I.V. fluid (perhaps 2–3 liters for 1st hour depending on blood pressure and pulse).

2. Monitor urinary output (mannitol may be given to promote urination).

3. Digitalis may be given in cases where heart failure is a possibility.

4. Possible administration of medication to increase cardiac output (if needed).

5. Oxygen may be given.

6. Other procedures as necessary may be used.

7. Continue to monitor kidney and brain functions, and vital signs.

Figure 5.3 represents a flowchart which summarizes how the various heat related illnesses can result from heat stress. It is important for the readers to realize that once the athlete undergoes a bout of heat exhaustion or heat stroke, he/she may have damaged their thermoregulatory system. The thermoregulatory system has a set point of 37°C, but the damaged thermoregulatory system may have a higher set point and thus the athlete may become more susceptible to bouts of heat related illness and can further damage the thermoregulatory system. Therefore, it is important for the athlete to exercise preventive measures in order to reduce the chances of heat related illnesses.

FURTHER GENERAL READING

Barr, S.I., et al. (1990). Fluid Replacement During Prolonged Exercise: Effects of Water, Saline, or No Fluid, *Med. Sci. Sports Exerc.* 23:811–817.

Coyle, E.F., et al. (1983). Carbohydrate Feeding During Prolonged Strenuous Exercise Can Delay Fatigue, *J. of Appl. Phys.* 55:230–235.

Kirkendall, D.T. (1993). Effects of Nutrition on Performance in Soccer, *Med. Sci. Sports Exerc.* 25:1370–1374.

Chapter

I *SIX*

Adaptation to Endurance Training

Endurance training connotes a process of adaptive changes to achieve the strength, power, and cardiorespiratory capacity necessary in order to complete a specific physical task. Endurance training requires several months of rhythmic and continued exercise, and results in an increase in the body's number of capillaries, maximal oxygen uptake, stroke volume, and muscle enzymes. Moreover, endurance training increases the sectional size of slow type fibers. There can also be an actual conversion of fast type fibers Type IIB (Type 2B) to fast Type IIA (Type 2A) to slow Type I. The Type IIB fibers are capable of lasting longer than the Type IIA fibers while Type I fibers are slow and long lasting like those of a marathon runner. Therefore, there are major underlying biochemical changes in the various organs and cells involved in the physical activity that provides the needed energy, strength and power to carry out specific tasks. Soccer requires a combination of slow and fast fibers because playing soccer is a combination of quick actions lasting less than 1–2 minutes and prolonged activities which can last 5–10 minutes.

Understanding endurance training has become a very serious scientific endeavor. In the past twenty years, there has been an increase in our understanding of the physiology and biochemistry of exercise. There has also been an increase in interest in the mechanism of how exercise induces physiological and biochemical adaptation at the cellular and organ level and how this accounts for the improved performance of athletes in a given sport. In an oversimplified way, we can view exercise as a transient damage to the tissue that stimulates repair beyond the original level. In this context, a prolonged resting period between bouts of exercise is essential for full repair of muscle tissue.

Endurance in sports means the ability of the person to perform a specific prolonged exercise or type of work, in order to achieve a reasonable goal without adverse reactions such as fatigue, exhaustion, or injury. Endurance can mean different things for different tasks (ex. sport activity), as each task may involve unique muscle groups and skill levels. Therefore, there are several components of endurance that develop differentially during repetitive endurance training for a specific sport. The components which contribute to increased endurance are: **muscle strength and power, the cardiovascular system, and the respiratory system**. Cardio-respiratory endurance requires varying intensities in different sports. However, strength and power can vary in magnitude from muscle to muscle. Therefore, local or regional muscle group endurance is quite important for a given sport. During an endurance training period consisting of repetitive exercise for several months, the muscles adapt to generate force and to maintain a supply of energy. The key factor in endurance training is the exertion of physical stress with certain frequency and for variable lengths of time. This chronic muscular activity stimulates growth of the muscle as well as the development of endurance in terms of oxygen delivery, energy production, and permanent metabolic and structural changes. Therefore, endurance training in this context is a low level, prolonged intensity, aerobic training type of exercise where the system can utilize oxygen as the initial trigger of energy source. In general, the first aspect of endurance adaptation is the adaptation of the cardiovascular/respiratory system to accommodate the increased demand for oxygen uptake and delivery.

CARDIOVASCULAR/RESPIRATORY ADAPTATION

Rhythmic and continued exercise requires a greater use of oxygen at the muscle site. Therefore, the routes of uptake and transport of oxygen from the air to muscle tissues must adapt to the increased rate of delivery and extraction. A measurement of cardiorespiratory endurance is the VO_{2max}. VO_{2max}, which differs from person to person, is a measurement of the maximal oxygen uptake during the maximal exercise. In order to compare exercise-related data from person to person, the data are expressed relative to a specific level of intensity of exercise and expressed as a percent of VO_{2max}. To illustrate its importance, endurance training can change the VO_{2max} by as much as 20%. This is the first indication that true structural and biochemical changes must occur in order to metabolize the increased oxygen uptake. The first apparent result of exercise is the immediate increase in heart rate. The average resting heart rate is about 80 beats per min; however, during exercise the heart rate can go as high as 190 beats per min. After several months of endurance training heart rates in resting states can go as low as 40 beats per min. This reflects several factors of adaptation to exercise, one of them being the autonomic nervous system. However, despite the lowered heart rate, the heart still provides a greater cardiac output. This is because the volume of blood pumped per beat or stroke volume increases by as much as 80%. In a highly trained athlete, the refilling of the heart with return blood is more complete. More importantly, the left ventricle strength and power is dramatically increased. The left ventricle undergoes hypertrophy with endurance training, due to increased heart muscle mass and volume. Heart size is greater in an endurance trained athlete by as much as 25%, as compared to a sedentary person. Moreover, the amount of contractile proteins is increased and the composition of these contractile proteins are changed. Also, oxygen delivery of the blood supply to the heart is improved because the number and size of capillaries per cross-sectional area of muscle increases by as much as 50% due to endurance training. Endurance training also improves (by as much as 80%) the muscle content of myoglobin, a protein which carries oxygen within the muscle tissue. These dramatic biochemical adaptations in the oxygen delivery system parallels those of the heart and thus complements the entire scope of the biochemical adaptation which results in a better performance by the trained athlete.

BLOOD VOLUME AND COMPOSITION

There are three major changes in the blood due to endurance training: (1) increased blood volume; (2) increased hematocrit (i.e., increase in the total number of red blood cells (RBCs)); and (3) decreased blood viscosity. The increased blood volume is as high as 20%. However, the increase in RBC mass is less pronounced and as a consequence the viscosity of the blood decreases. The increase in blood volume is of primary importance for the endurance trained athlete. The increased blood volume enhances O_2 delivery as well as enhancing microcirculation (i.e., small capillaries within muscle). The increase in microcirculation is even more pronounced due to the blood's reduced viscosity. The trained athlete also has another advantage in the greater capacity to clear lactate from the muscle and utilize lactate as an energy substrate. Thus, the level of blood lactate in a trained athlete is lower than that of the sedentary person. This phenomenon is referred to as the lactate shift.

A trained athlete, therefore, has greater endurance with less fatigue and cramps due to decreased levels of blood lactate.

ENERGY SOURCE

The direct energy source in cells is adenosine triphosphate (ATP). ATP is produced by the mitochondrial (the mitochondria is the powerhouse of the cell) enzymes. The Krebs cycle utilizes oxygen (an aerobic process) (also referred to it as oxidation) in the production of ATP. In order to utilize larger amounts of oxygen to produce more and more ATP for the trained athlete, the number of mitochondria increases by over 100% and the size of each mitochondria increases by as much as 35%. Therefore, there is a concomitant increase in all of the enzymes involved. A trained athlete develops the ability to store in skeletal muscle a greater amount of glycogen (up to 40% more) and triglycerides (a type of fat) (1.8%) than an untrained one. Another advantage for a trained athlete is the increased ability to utilize free fatty acids by as much as 30%. This increase in free fatty acids use results in sparing glycogen for later use if needed. The increased use of free fatty acids is consistent with the increased fatty acid oxidation enzymes in the endurance trained athlete.

MUSCLE FIBER COMPOSITION

The motor unit is considered the terminal functional element responsible for movement. Even though the distinctions among the three types of units is somewhat arbitrary, they serve as an initial handle in understanding the complex number of muscles involved in endurance training induced adaptation. The "type 1" fibers are also called "slow/relaxing" or slow twitch. The "type 2" fibers are also called "fast/relaxing" or fast twitch. Type 2 fibers are classified into two major classes: type 2A and type 2B. Type 2B fibers "tend" (not in all cases) to represent the fast glycolytic (FG) (indicating quick utilization of glucose and stored glycogen during anaerobic process) and type 2A "tend" (not in all cases) to represent the fast oxidative-glycolytic (FOG) (indicating the utilization of oxidative process of Krebs cycle during aerobic process). There are also type 2C fibers that are considered intermediate between type 1 and type 2. Endurance exercise causes changes from type 2B to type 2A to type 1 (i.e., towards slower and more long lasting fibers) with concomitant changes in the amount of enzymes. Endurance training also causes changes in the calcium regulatory enzymes in order to accommodate the new type of fibers.

The adaptive process due to endurance training continues for up to six months beyond which little change occurs (see Figures 6.1 and 6.2). The cardiorespiratory parameters (VO_2, number of capillaries, enzymes), all increase in parallel in response to endurance training. However, increases in the muscle fiber conversion and the cross-sectional size occurs in a shorter time period (i.e., 1–2 months). Unfortunately, an absence of training results in a rapid decline of increased parameters to near control levels in 1–3 months. One exception may be the decline in the VO_2 and number of capillaries; in these cases, the decline is slower and may take about six months.

Soccer is a mixture of anaerobic and aerobic activities that requires endurance training and the use of slow fibers, and quick bursts of activity that requires anaerobic training and the use of fast fibers. In order to adapt the soccer player's muscles for the game, the athlete must consistently train both aerobically and anaerobically for prolonged periods of time.

It is fortunate that once adaptation is achieved, the maintenance program is much less rigorous than the adaptation program. It appears that to induce adaptation in muscle cells, the intensity, frequency and duration of training should be high compared to maintenance. Once endurance is achieved, the maintenance program can be as low as 40% of the intensity, frequency and duration without a loss in endurance. This is important for young athletes since most of them do not play soccer during the summer. Therefore, to maintain their achieved level of fitness and endurance, athletes must perform

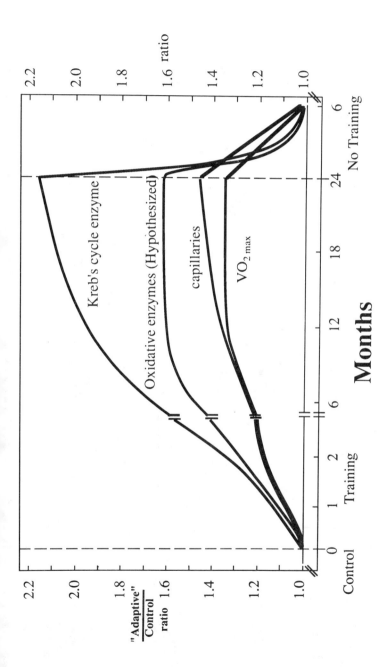

Figure 6.1. A schematic representation of the ratio of adaptation to control in man due to exercise based on data and hypothetical considerations for illustrative purposes. The figure is reproduced with permission from the publisher and the authors, Saltin et al., *Ann. N.Y. Acad. Sci.* 301:3–29, 1977. The curve on oxidative enzymes (hypothesized) was made by the authors.

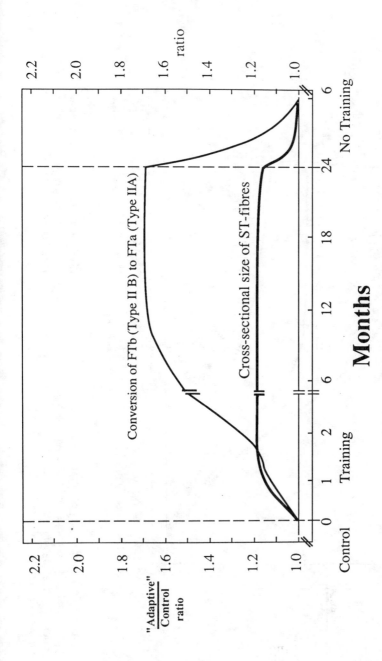

Figure 6.2. A schematic representation of the ratio of adaptation to control in man due to exercise based on data and hypothetical considerations for illustrative purposes. The figure is reproduced with permission from the publisher and the authors, Saltin et al., *Ann. N.Y. Acad. Sci.* 301:3–29, 1977.

a minimum of 2–3 workouts per week, consisting of 30–40 minutes of actually playing soccer or jogging and sprinting.

FURTHER GENERAL READING

Anderson, K.L. (1968). The Cardiovascular System in Exercise, in: *Exerc. Phys.*, ed. H.B. Falls, Academic Press, New York, USA.

Kjellberg, S., et al. (1949). Increase of the Amount of Hemoglobin and Blood Volume in Connection with Physical Training, *Acta Physiol. Cand.* 19:146.

Klug, G.A., and Tibbits, G.F. (1988). The Effect of Activity on Calcium Mediated Entry in Striated Muscle, *Exerc. Sports Sci. Rev.* 16:1–59.

McArdle, W.D., et al. (1991). *Exercise Physiology*, 3rd ed., pp. 1–853. Lea & Febiger, Philadelphia (USA).

Saltin, B., et al. (1977). Fiber Types and Metabolic Potentials of Skeletal Muscles in Sedentary Man and Endurance Runners, *Ann. N.Y. Acad. Sci.*, 301:3–29.

Wilmore, J.H., and Costill, D.L. (1988). Training For Sport and Activity, 3rd ed., pp. 1–420, Wm. C. Brown Publishers, Dubuque, Iowa (USA).

Chapter

SEVEN

Nutritional Requirement for Soccer Players

The most beneficial diet for a young soccer player involves eating balanced meals consisting of an average ratio of 5:1:1. of carbohydrates; proteins; fats. When exercising, the body primarily requires additional calories, and the best calories for an athlete to consume are in the form of carbohydrates. Increased exercise requires a proportional increase in the intake of carbohydrates. The pre-game meals should be primarily composed of carbohydrates, and balanced meals should be eaten prior to game days. Just prior to and during the game, the player should drink adequate amounts of cold water (2–3 glasses). In an ideal situation, the athlete should drink 4–6 ounces of water every 15–20 minutes.

Table 7.1. Estimated Amount of Carbohydrates, Proteins, and Fats a Soccer Player Should Ingest Daily

	Average activity			Endurance activity (2-hr soccer session*)		
	Player's weight			Player's weight		
	35 kg (77 lb)	55 kg (121 lb)	70 kg (154 lb)	35 kg (77 lb)	55 kg (121 lb)	70 kg (154 lb)
Carbohydrates (g)	200–400	315–630	400–600	350–450	550–707	700–900
Proteins (g)	40–45	60–70	80–90	40–45	60–70	80–90
Fats (g)	40–50	60–80	80–100	40–50	60–80	80–100

*It is estimated that a 1-hr intense soccer session consumes 550 calories. However, this number is much lower for a youth soccer session depending on age and intensity.

The human body is an organism which is composed of cells. Nutritional requirements are needed to maintain the normal cell functions in order to carry out the tasks which the body performs.

Like the rest of us, athletes, trainers, and coaches have a very limited knowledge of nutrition. Unfortunately, the societal pressures for winning induces athletes and others to invent the most bizarre concoctions of food which are then deemed proper "nutrition." These wild recipes are based on the most unscientific and the least documented studies. Most of these recipes are based on personal experiences associated with the food last eaten before a successful performance. For an athlete, a balanced diet should consist of three main constituents; carbohydrates, proteins, and fats, with a weight ratio of 5:1:1 (and a caloric ratio of about 3:1:1) (see Table 7.1). Unfortunately, the current average American diet is composed of a weight ratio of 3:1:1 (with a caloric ratio of about 2:1:1). In other words, there is too much intake of fats and proteins and not enough intake of carbohydrates. Healthy and balanced nutritional intake by the individual will not only help the athlete but also will diminish the chances of developing coronary heart disease and becoming obese.

CARBOHYDRATES

Carbohydrates are composed of carbon, hydrogen, and oxygen. The simplest form of carbohydrate is the sugar glucose. Other examples of simple carbohydrates are fructose and galactose. Examples of some complex carbohydrates are starch (e.g., from potatoes, pasta, fruits and vegetables, bread, bagels, cereal and rice) and cellulose (a source of dietary fiber). The average American currently consumes 50% of carbohydrates as simple sugars, mainly in the form of sucrose. However, sucrose causes a fluctuation in insulin secretion. Too much insulin in the blood may lead to low blood sugar (hypoglycemia). Low blood sugar could contribute to symptoms such as weakness, dizziness, and hunger sensations. None of these symptoms are beneficial to the athletes during their activities. Fructose (fruit sugar) is absorbed well in the intestine and does not stimulate insulin secretion. Thus it does not promote large fluctuations of blood sugar levels. As we have mentioned earlier, exercise suppresses insulin secretion. Therefore, sugar intake during exercise will not lead to low blood sugar.

Carbohydrates serve as the main source of energy for the body, and they also serve as an important source of metabolic by-products. These byproducts are critical for many cell functions including protein sparing, fat utilization, and energy production.

1. **Protein Sparing.** Proteins, as we will see later, are the main building blocks needed for muscle maintenance, repair, and growth. Proteins can also serve as a source of energy when carbohydrates are low. When needed, glucose is actually formed from proteins as is the case in marathon running or any other prolonged exercise (greater than 90 minutes). Under these conditions, muscle proteins are degraded in order to provide a source of glucose. This actually causes a reduction in muscle content and in the process increases the concentration of nitrogen (from the degradation of proteins) excreted in the urine. Therefore, the maintenance of an adequate supply of carbohydrates or body stores of carbohydrates in the form of glycogen is important in reducing muscle breakdown.

2. **Carbohydrates as a Primer for Fat Utilization.** Carbohydrates in the body undergo metabolism (i.e., breakdown

to smaller units) in order to release useful energy. Some of the breakdown products of carbohydrates are needed to break down fats and release their energy. Therefore, when insufficient carbohydrates exist, fatty acid breakdown becomes incomplete, which results in acidic body fluids; this is not conducive for normal function.

3. **Carbohydrates as a Source of Fuel for the Brain.** The brain (i.e., central nervous system) almost solely utilizes glucose as its source of energy. Under low carbohydrates conditions, the brain utilizes larger amounts of fats as a source of energy. Nevertheless, low blood glucose due to even modestly low carbohydrate levels could cause the symptoms of hypoglycemia mentioned earlier, and under extreme conditions could even cause irreversible brain damage. However, the brain can adapt by using fats as a source of energy within a week of experiencing low blood sugar.

4. **Exercise and Stored Energy.** Glucose and carbohydrates are the most likely sources of energy when there is an immediate demand, such as in anaerobic exercise (e.g., sprinting). However, endurance sports are aerobic in nature and they utilize the most efficient forms of metabolism (using oxygen) to break down sugar and carbohydrates which are then used as energy sources.

A carbohydrate-rich diet results in increased stores of muscle and liver glycogen. About 75% of glycogen is usually stored in muscle, about 20% in liver, and the remainder is stored in the blood. Glycogen stores are the critical factor that determines how long an athlete can exercise before becoming exhausted. There is a near linear relationship between the length of time an athlete can sustain an exercise, and the amount of stored glycogen which is used. Soccer players have been reported to be less energetic during the second half of play due to glycogen depletion in muscles. The ingestion of glucose polymers (series of glucose molecules hooked together) during exercise can prolong the exercise time to exhaustion. Moreover, glucose-polymers do not decrease the transit time of food in the intestine. The decrease in transit time in intestine would decrease absorption of the glucose-polymer. After an event, soccer players, just as other athletes, have low levels of muscle glycogen. Therefore, it is advisable for the athlete to ingest large quantities of carbohydrates within the first two hours after a game or practice. The muscle content of glycogen is very low following an event and thus there is an enhanced ability in the muscle to store glycogen. Soccer players should have high levels of muscle glycogen content before the game. Since the glycogen storage enzymes work much more efficiently after exercise, it is important that the athlete takes advantages of this enhanced proficiency by ingesting a large amount of carbohydrates after a game. In this way, the player will build up an adequate store of carbohydrates which can then be utilized at subsequent games. Obviously, adequate rest and proper food intake must accompany exercise.

PROTEINS

Proteins consist of carbon, oxygen, hydrogen, and nitrogen. Nitrogen is the distinct atom that is associated with proteins as compared to fats and carbohydrates which only consist of carbon, oxygen, and hydrogen. Also, proteins may contain sulfur, phosphorus, and iron. Proteins, which are large molecules made up of smaller molecules called amino acids, are required for numerous bodily functions. Among the most important body functions that involves proteins are: enzymatic processes; transport; storage; the delivery of small molecules such as iron (Fe^{2+}), sodium (Na^+), potassium (K^+), calcium (Ca^{2+}) etc; muscle function (e.g., in skeletal and heart muscle); mechanical support (e.g., collagen in fibers); the immune system (all antibodies against foreign invaders are proteins); nerve function (e.g., many neurotransmitters are proteins); and growth and differentiation (e.g., hormones, regulation of genes, etc). There are nine amino acids (called essential amino acids) which are not synthesized in the adult body, and must be provided through the intake of foods. The other eleven amino acids are synthesized in the body and thus need not be provided by a food source. These are called *nonessential amino acids*. The most important sources of proteins are meat, fish, poultry, eggs, and dairy products.

At the beginning of each heavy training season, serious athletes should increase their intake of proteins by almost 20–30%.

This increased protein intake will compensate for the immediate need to increase muscle mass, and other amino acid-requiring proteins such as red blood cells and myoglobin (the oxygen carrier in muscle). As we have mentioned earlier, it has been observed that prolonged exercise causes protein breakdown when carbohydrate reserves are low. Therefore, an athlete should have an abundance of glycogen stores in the muscles in order to prevent muscle wastage and to maintain peak performance levels. Glycogen stores are replenished by the intake of a sufficient amount of carbohydrates.

FATS

Fats, like carbohydrates, also consist of carbon, oxygen and hydrogen. Also, fats may contain phosphorous, nitrogen and other elements. Fats are required for numerous bodily functions; among the most important are: (1) energy stores (i.e., fats produce the energy currency of the body, ATP); (2) structure (e.g., all cell membranes are made of fats); (3) hormones (some are derived from fats); (4) intracellular messengers; (5) insulation (e.g., fats prevent body heat loss); and (6) vitamin delivery (fat-soluble vitamins such as A, D, E, and K are carried by fats through the bloodstream).

Almost all fats which are required for bodily functions can be synthesized in the body, with linoleic acid being the only possible exception. Therefore, the concept of essential versus non-essential fats is not as well defined as for amino acids. However as mentioned earlier, fat intake is needed for the absorption of fat-soluble vitamins. Fats are derived from meat, fish, poultry, and dairy products (e.g., butter).

In moderate exercise, energy is equally derived from carbohydrates and fats. During longer exercises (1 hr), carbohydrate resources are depleted, and fat utilization increases to up to 80% of all energy required. Endurance athletes can utilize more fats at an earlier stage of exercise, and thus can save carbohydrates for later use. The use of caffeine also increases early use of fats as a source of energy.

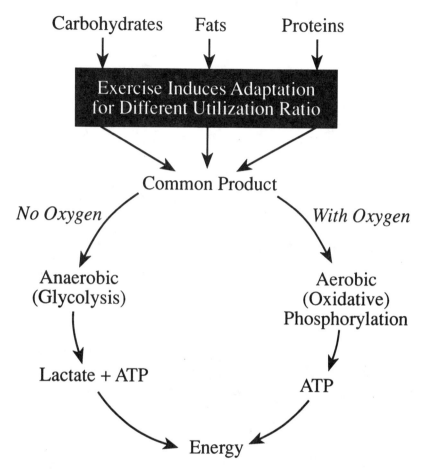

Figure 7.1. Flowchart of the metabolic pathways for foodstuff to energy production.

WATER AND ELECTROLYTES (see Chapter 5)

Figure 7.1 summarizes the use of foodstuffs as a source of energy under aerobic and anaerobic conditions. Furthermore, the figure shows that exercise causes adaptation in the utilization of different amounts of the three sources of nutrition.

Drugs and hormones similarly influence the ratio of utilization of these three sources of energy.

FURTHER GENERAL READING

Jones, M., and Pedoe, T. (1989). Blood Doping: A Literature Review, _Brit. J. of Sports Med._ 23:84–88.

Medical Commission of the International Olympic Committee (1989). _Brit. J. of Sports Med._ 23:60.

O'Neil, F., et al. (1986). Research and Applications of Current Topics in Sports Nutrition, _J. of the Am. Dietetic Ass._ 86:1007–1015.

Inge, K., and Garden, L. (1990). Nutrition Advice for Athletes, _Aust. Fam. Phy._ 19:133–138.

Kirkendall, D.T. (1993). Effects of Nutrition on Performance in Soccer, _Med. Sci. Sports Exerc._ 25:1370–1374.

Chapter
EIGHT

Drugs and Hormones in Sport

Unfortunately, there is a widespread use of drugs and hormones among athletes in order to try to enhance the accomplishment of short range goals. Examples of such drugs and hormones used are: steroids; growth hormones; amphetamines; and, the most seemingly benign of all of them, caffeine. Anabolic steroids in males (androgens or "male hormones") can cause stunted growth, testicular atrophy, liver damage, and increased breast size. In females, use of these same steroids can lead to male pattern baldness, deepening of the voice, unwanted hair patterns, enlargement of the clitoris, and dysfunction of the reproductive system and menstrual cycle. Growth hormone use can cause gigantism if given before the end of puberty, and can contribute to skin abnormalities, and enlarged bones. Amphetamine use can lead to addiction, headache, dizziness, confusion, anxiety, aggressiveness, impaired judgment, and may ultimately cause death. Caffeine use can spare carbohydrate depletion by the increased use of fats. However, because caffeine is a central stimulant, its heavy use can cause headaches, anxiety, insomnia, and increased urine output which can contribute to dehydration.

Athletes have always searched for a competitive edge over others using numerous ergogenic aids. The term "ergogenic aid" connotes any agent (e.g., physical or nutritional etc.) that enhances performance. Great athletes have combined natural abilities, rigorous training, good coaching, and an outstanding competitive nature which enable them to achieve their competitive edge. Unfortunately, in modern times athletes have sought the use of biomedical knowledge about drugs and hormones in order to seek an unfair advantage. Aside from the unethical and illegal nature of the use of these drugs and hormones in sports, it is often dangerous to the athlete's own health and competitive edge. Moreover, these drugs, in addition to being dangerous, are illegal to use. Also, there is little documented scientific evidence that some of these drugs enhance performance. Therefore, the individual can significantly risk his/her health for an unsubstantiated and most likely detrimental effect of these drugs.

The following drugs and hormones will be discussed: steroids; growth hormones; amphetamines; and caffeine.

STEROIDS

The various types of steroids are either naturally occurring physiological steroid hormones or their synthetic analogues. All steroid hormones are derived from cholesterol. The relevant steroids about which the athlete should be aware of are called androgens. They produce an androgenic as well as an anabolic effect on the body. Androgenic effects are those effects which are related to male sexual maturation, and anabolic effects are those effects related to growth, such as an increase in mass and the rate of bone and muscle maturation.

The aim of synthetic steroids is to have compounds that selectively enhance anabolic effects without any androgenic effects. This is especially critical for female users. Heavy and prolonged steroid users can suffer from stunted growth due to early closure of the growth plates, liver damage, testicular atrophy, increased breast size (in males), and an increased risk of cardiovascular diseases.

Athletes use steroids to increase muscle mass and strength. Although there may be some evidence that steroids users have a greater muscle mass, the mechanism of increased muscle mass due to steroids use is not yet clear. Unfortunately, steroid users may gain some advantage in certain sports competitions; however, the risks far outweigh the benefits. Direct effects of steroids on muscle are controversial. It is thought that steroids use enhances the desire for more training and the ability to sustain more pain, in addition to a direct increase in muscle mass. Therefore, it is thought that steroids act on the brain in a way which results in the desire for more frequent training that contributes to the eventual increase in muscle mass.

GROWTH HORMONE (GH)

GH is a naturally occurring hormone which is secreted by the pituitary gland. GH is involved in tissue growth by enhancing protein synthesis. Subsequently, this leads to an increased muscle mass and increased utilization of fats (for fuel), which spares carbohydrates. The fact that GH occurs naturally in the body is very attractive to athletes because they incorrectly assume that it is safe. However, prolonged and heavy use of GH in unphysiological quantities increases the risk of gigantism, skin abnormalities, oversized soft tissues, and enlarged bones. A further danger associated with the prolonged use of exogenous GH is the depression of physiological GH secretion. This decrease in normal physiological GH secretion can cause deleterious effects.

In addition, certain amino acids can temporarily enhance GH release. However, there is no strong evidence that the long-term use of GH decreases body fat and increases muscle mass.

AMPHETAMINES

Amphetamines are prescription drugs which act as stimulants (also called "uppers") of the central nervous system (i.e., brain). Amphetamines reduce the sense of fatigue due to heavy exercise. The decrease in the sense of fatigue due to amphetamines is dangerous in itself because it inhibits our bodies' sense of when to slow down or stop a given exercise. Amphetamines also increase the following; vasoconstriction, blood sugar, pulse rate, breathing rate, and muscle tension. Amphetamines, therefore, act like the "fight and flight" hormones, epinephrine and norepinephrine. The perception of enhanced performance in a specific sport, however, is not supported by the research data. The undocumented enhancement of performance due to amphetamines could lead to the deleterious side effects of the drug. The dangers associated with the use of amphetamines include; addiction, headaches, dizziness, confusion, increased reaction time, impaired judgement, anxiety, aggressiveness, insomnia, and possibly death with heavy usage.

CAFFEINE

Caffeine (methylxanthine) is a mild stimulant of the central nervous system. Caffeine is a natural component of coffee, tea, chocolate, etc. and acts as a stimulant to reduce the sense of fatigue due to exercise. Caffeine also increases the use of fats as fuel and thus spares carbohydrates which leads to added endurance for the athlete. Also, caffeine can increase the VO_{2max}; in addition, there is a small direct effect on the increased force of muscle contraction. Furthermore, caffeine can increase the availability of cellular calcium to the muscle. However, there are conflicting reports on the effect of caffeine on various physiological factors. Because caffeine is a stimulant, its use is associated with the following side effects; headaches, increased anxiety, insomnia, and increased urine output (diuresis) which can contribute to the dehydration of the athlete when exercising in a hot environment.

FURTHER GENERAL READING

McNaughton, L. (1987). Two Levels of Caffeine Ingestion on Blood Lactate and Free Fatty Acid Responses During Incremental Exercise, *Res. Quar. for Exer. and Sport.* 58(3):255–259.

Weir, J., et al. (1987). A High Carbohydrate Diet Negates the Metabolic Effects of Caffeine During Exercise, *Med. Sci. Sports Exer.* 19:100–105.

Sutton, J., and Lazarus, L. (1976). Growth Hormone in Exercise: Comparison of Physiological and Pharmacological Stimuli, *J. Appl. Physiol.* 41:523–527.

Crist, D.M., et al. (1983). Effects of Androgen-Anabolic Steroids on Neuromuscular Power and Body Composition, *J. Appl. Physiol. Respir. Environ. Exer. Physiol.* 54(2):366–370.

Haupt, H.A., and Rovere, G.D. (1984). Anabolic Steroids: A Review of the Literature, *Am. J. Sports Med.* 12:469–484.

Lenders, J.W. (1988). Deleterious Effects of Analogic Steroids on Serum Lipoproteins, Blood Pressure, and Liver Function in Amateur Body Builders, *Int. J. of Sports Med.* 9(1):19–23.

Wilson, J.D., and Griffin, J.E. (1980). The Use and Misuse of Androgens, *Metab.* 29:1278–1295.

American Academy of Orthopedic Surgeons (1991). *Athletic Training and Sports Medicine*, 2nd ed., American Academy of Orthopedic Surgeons, Park Ridge, Illinois.

Chapter

NINE

Gender Differences and Skill Development

Recent evidence indicates that elite female athletes are catching up with elite male athletes. This new evidence supports the conviction among some people that the differences in athletic performances between the two genders are primarily due to outdated societal expectations and values. However, despite this new evidence, there are important physiological and biochemical differences that could contribute to different growths in skills and performance between males and females for a given sport. For example, the onset of puberty is about 2 years earlier in girls than in boys. Because of this, girls height and weight is different from that of boys. Males usually have larger mass and greater aerobic power than females. However, puberty can also contribute to the delay in the acquisition of skills since skills are dependent on a sense of coordination coupled with the height and weight of the individual. Finally, female athletes may experience athletic amenorrhea (i.e., absence of their menstrual period). Athletic amenorrhea is associated with; low body fat, heavy exercise, poor nutrition, and genetic differences that influences the athlete's susceptibility to menstrual dysfunction.

There are obviously numerous physiological and biochemical differences between males and females. The real question is: are those physiological and biochemical differences the basis for some of the differences in performance in sports among males and females?

This is a highly controversial area. There are no clear cut answers at this time. The complicating factor has been that the societal expectations for performance in sports have been skewed in the past, (including the recent past) towards males. It is this important social factor that cannot be discounted when males outperform females in certain sports. However, the most recent research data indicates that the differences between genders is shrinking and this argues against inherent differences in abilities. Further support for this argument comes from the fact that present day elite female athletes in certain athletic events perform equal to or better than elite male athletes of just ten years ago.

Despite the above disclaimers in gender differences in athletic performance, there are important physiological, biochemical, and performance differences that have to be taken into consideration and dealt with in order to improve coaching and performance outcome in sports for both genders. We should note, however, that these differences between genders are insignificant before adolescence (puberty).

HEIGHT AND WEIGHT

In the first two years of adolescence, there is a high rate of growth in height and weight for both genders. Usually a girl's growth stops around 16 1/2 years old, and boy's growth stops around 18 years old. As we have mentioned in the summary, the onset of puberty is about 2 years earlier in girls than boys.

Therefore, girls obtain full maturity of their bones earlier than boys. Bone growth is faster and more fully developed when it is subjected to exercise (i.e., moderate physical stress), as exercise is important for the tensile strength and diameter of the bone. The primary sites that determine height are at the growth plates (epiphyses) of the femur (upper leg). Therefore, proper treatment of injuries to growth plates is important in preventing the premature closure of these plates which can result in shorter stature.

MUSCLE

In both males and females, the mechanism of muscle adaptation due to exercise in terms of energy producing enzymes, fiber composition, and oxygen delivery, is the same. Full strength is fully attained at the age of 20 for females and between the ages of 20–30 in males. However, in males there is an increase in muscle mass due to testosterone (a male hormone). Females have much lower testosterone levels than males, but they secrete estrogen which enhances fat deposition in breasts and hips. Estrogen secretion does not increase muscle mass. When males combine strength training with their increased muscle mass, they can obtain greater upper and lower body strength than females. Moreover, strength is related not only to the muscle mass but also to the neuromuscular status and the ability to recruit more fibers by the nervous system. As we mentioned earlier, there are no gender differences in aerobic parameters. If the aerobic power parameter VO_{2max} is expressed per weight, both genders have similar values. However, because males have larger mass, the overall aerobic output is greater.

SKILLS

The acquisition of skills begins at birth and continues throughout life. Skills are dependent on the continued development of the neuromotor system. Skill also requires the coordination of the sense known as the perceptomotor system, which consists of the coordination of visual kinesthetic, and auditory senses. Attainment of skills requires storage of learned information which depends on the continued repetition of the correct function. The development of the nervous system plays a critical role in skill development. At early stages of life nerve myelination (insulation of the nerve from the environment in order to conduct nerve impulses efficiently) is incomplete. This incomplete myelination results in slower nerve conduction and therefore less coordination than that of adults. At puberty both males and females experience a high rate of growth in height and weight, and development of neuromotor function.

Clumsiness is a fact of life with a prepubescent child. During this normal developmental period, the brain has to continuously adjust to the increased neuromotor function, as well as to the new spatial positions of the extremities (i.e., toes and fingers due to increased limb length). This hypothesis of the brain re-learning limb lengths can explain the clumsiness experienced during adolescence. There is data showing that males have a slight advantage in certain skills. However, more recent data on the same types of skills indicate that these differences are becoming smaller and smaller. This argues for social factors in skill levels of the two genders rather than inherent differences in the body physiology and biochemistry.

ATHLETIC AMENORRHEA

Athletic amenorrhea is the absence of the menstrual period for a length of time (e.g., greater than one year), and is associated with heavy exercise. Athletic amenorrhea is also strongly associated with the malfunction of the hypothalamus. The hypothalamus manufactures and secretes gonadotropin-releasing hormone (GnRH) in order to stimulate the pituitary gland which in turn releases follicle-stimulating hormone (FSH) and luteinizing hormone (LH). Both of these gonadotropins are involved in maintaining a normal menstrual cycle.

In the general population, the occurrence of amenorrhea averages about 5%; however, among heavy dedicated athletes it increases to 20 to 50%. For unknown reasons, ballet dancers and runners have a higher incidence of athletic amenorrhea than other athletes. There is evidence that athletic amenorrhea is associated with a decrease in GnRH release from the hypothalamus. There are several factors that may contribute to athletic amenorrhea:

(1) Low body fat (below 17%). However, there are athletes with body fat well below 17% who have normal menstrual cycles

(2) exercise-induced increase in the secretion of brain endorphins (natural morphine-like proteins in the body) such as opiates, which can inhibit GnRH secretion.

(3) exercise-induced increase in the secretion of melatonin from the brain. Melatonin can decrease GnRH secretion.

There are numerous factors contributing to athletic amenorrhea, and, more importantly, there is an interplay among these factors which contributes to the frequency of the disorder. The contributing factors include; delayed puberty, stress (physical or emotional), poor nutrition (especially anorexia and bulimia), low body fat, heavy training (especially when combined with poor nutrition), genetic influence, and hormonal dysfunction. Amenorrhea can contribute to osteoporosis (decreased bone density), and the eventual loss of bone mass. Most symptoms of athletic amenorrhea are reversed when the factors contributing to amenorrhea cease to exist. However, there may not be a full recovery of bone mass. Therefore, if there is a delayed menarche (onset of menstrual cycle) or amenorrhea, the athlete should see her physician to determine which (if any) of these factors may be involved in her particular case.

FURTHER GENERAL READING

Colley and Beech (1988). *Advances in Psychology. Cognition and Action in Skilled Behavior,* Elsevier Science Publishers, pp. 273–331.

Haywood, K. (1989). *Life Span Motor Development,* Human Kinetics Publishers, Inc.

Keogh, et al. (1990). *Movement Skill Development,* Macmillan Publishing Company.

Whipp, B.J., and Ward, S.A. (1992). Will Women Soon Outrun Men? *Nature* 235:25.

Smyth and Wing (1984). *The Psychology of Human Movement*, Academic Press, Inc., pp. 215–240.

Glass, A., et al. (1987). Amenorrhea in Olympic Marathon Runners, *Fertility and Sterility* 48:740–745.

Henley K., et al. (1988). Exercise-Induced Menstrual Dysfunction, *Ann. Rev. Med.* 39:443–451.

Jones, K.P., et al. (1985). Comparison of Bone Density in Amenorrheic Woman Due to Athletics, Weight Loss, and Premature Menopause, *Obstetrics and Gynecology* 66:5–8.

Kaiserauer, S., et al. (1988). Nutritional, Physiological, and Menstrual Status of Distance Runner, *Med. and Sci. in Sports and Exer.* 21:120–129.

Loucks, A.B., et al. (1984). Exercise-Induced Stress Responses of Amenorrheic and Eumenorrheic Runners, *J. of Clin. Endocrin. and Metab.* 59:1109–1119.

White, C.M., et al. (1990). Amenorrhea, Osteopenia, and the Female Athlete, *Ped. Clinics of North Am.* 37(5):1125–1141.

Further General Reading

The following are the best general references for further reading. The reader can obtain a great deal more detailed knowledge from these books. However, they require some scientific background.

McArdle, W.D., et al. (1991). *Exercise Physiology*, 3rd ed., pp. 1–853. Lea & Febiger, Philadelphia (USA).

Wilmore, J.H., et al. (1988). *Training for Sport and Activity*, 3rd ed., pp. 1–420, Wm. C. Brown Publishers, Dubuque, Iowa (USA).

American College of Sports Medicine (1991). *Guidelines for Exercise Testing and Prescription*, 4th ed., pp. 1–314. Lea and Febiger, Philadelphia (USA).

Committee on Sports Medicine and Fitness (1991). *American Academy of Pediatrics, Sports Medicine: Health Care for Young Athlete*, 2nd ed. American Academy of Pediatrics, Elk Grove Village, IL (USA).

Harries et al., eds. (1994). *Oxford Textbook of Sports Medicine*. Oxford University Press, New York (USA).

GLOSSARY

achilles tendon: the tendon joining the calf (gastronomius) and (soleus muscles) of the leg to the bone of the heel.

acromioclavicular joint: a joint located at the top of the shoulder formed by the scapula and clavicle.

adductor muscle: a muscle that draws towards the midline of the body.

aerobic (exercise): when muscle contracts in the presence of oxygen.

amino acids: small organic compounds that are the building blocks for proteins. There are 20 amino acids.

amphetamines: chemicals that stimulate the central nervous system. Often used as street drugs which, when abused, can lead to psychosis, delusion, and in some cases, suicide. Street names for the drug include "pep pills," "speed," "ice," "black beauties," and "lid poppers."

anaerobic (exercise): when muscle contracts in the absence of oxygen. For example, in sprinting the muscles function faster than the delivery system can provide sufficient oxygen. Breakdown of carbohydrates without oxygen causes formation of lactic acid (lactate).

analgesic: relieving pain (i.e., with the use of a drug).

androgens: hormones that increase male characteristics.

anterior: toward the front frontal view, opposite to posterior.

anterior cruciate ligament: attaches the lateral side of the femur to the frontal side of the tibia.

apophysis: projection from a bone.

arthrodesis (also called ankylosis). This is a surgical procedure to relieve pain or provide more support.

athletic amenorrhea: an irregular menstrual cycle often associated with heavy exercise.

ATP (adenosine triphosphate): An organic molecule used as the most prevalent energy currency in all cells of the body. It contains three phosphates linked together. Breakdown of the terminal phosphate releases energy utilized in numerous cellular functions. ATP is the source of energy for muscles.

autonomic nervous system: part of the nervous system that regulates involuntary body functions such as skeletal and cardiac muscles, smooth muscle (intestine), and glands. The system consists of two parts — the sympathetic nervous system in charge of increased heart rate, vasoconstriction, and raising the blood pressure, and the parasympathetic nervous system in charge of slowing the heart rate, increasing intestinal movement, and increasing glandular function.

avulsion: an injury involving torn skin.

ballistic stretching: quick stretching of a muscle beyond its normal range. Not recommended.

blister: formation of a fluid-filled bubble which separates the skin from the underlying tissue.

blood pressure: hydrostatic pressure exerted by circulating blood against the walls of arteries.

blood volume: the volume of the entire blood in the body: about 5 liters for a 70-kg person.

bone scan: the use of a radioactive substance injected into a vein along with an imaging device to visualize bone structure and possible pathology.

brace: a device which holds and supports any part of the body in the correct position while allowing it to function.

bronchospasm: constriction of the air passages in the tracheobronchial tree.

caffeine: a chemical compound found in coffee and chocolate. Caffeine is a central nervous system stimulant.

calcaneus: the heel bone.

capillaries: small vessels that connect arteries and veins in tissues and muscles and allows the exchange of nutrients (e.g., oxygen and sugar) with waste products due to muscle activities.

carbohydrates: varied organic compounds such as saccharides and starches which serve as the main source of energy for the body.

Gum and cellulose are also carbohydrates, but humans lack the enzymes needed to digest them.

cardiovascular system: the heart and blood vessels. The heart pumps blood into vessels to deliver nutrients to muscles and tissues and removes waste products.

cartilage: a tough elastic connective tissue found in joints, the end of bones, nose, and ears.

cellulose: a specific kind of carbohydrate found in the cell walls of plants. The human body cannot digest cellulose.

charlie horse: a sudden and painful cramping of the quadriceps or hamstring muscles usually due to aggravation of damaged muscles by athletic activity.

circuit training: the use of several stations (10–15) for exercise that combines aerobic and strength training.

compartment syndrome: increased compression of an artery resulting in reduced blood flow. This is a serious pathology that could cause permanent damage to a hand or foot.

contusion: an injury to soft tissues without skin breakage.

cryotherapy: the use of cold temperature (i.e., ice) to lower metabolism in therapy of muscle injury.

dehydration: loss of water, a serious medical problem.

deltoid ligament: the medial ligament of the ankle which joins the medial malleolus with the talus.

digitalis: a long-used drug that strengthens the heart pump.

displaced fracture: a fracture of a limb associated with deformity.

distal: away from

dorsiflex: upward movement to the back (i.e., when the foot moves towards the shin).

economic training: using one exercise session to achieve multiple training purposes.

edema: excess fluid accumulation in tissue.

electrolytes: salts in solutions (i.e., body fluid) which dissociate into ions. For example, in such solution table salt dissociates into sodium ions (Na^+) and chloride ions (Cl^-). Body fluid electrolytes include Na^+, Cl^-, K^+, Mg^{2+}, Ca^{2+}, and others. The maintenance of certain concentrations of electrolytes inside versus outside the cell is critical in maintaining cell viability and function.

endorphins: chemical compounds (neuropeptides) secreted in the brain that have many effects on the body, e.g., feeling high and analgesia. Endorphins are released during exercise.

endurance: the ability of a person to perform a prolonged sporting event without adverse effects such as fatigue, exhaustion, or injury.

enzyme: a protein that catalyzes (speeds up) a reaction without being consumed.

epiphysis: the terminal end of a long bone.

ergogenic aids: any compounds or activity that enhance the ability to achieve greater work output.

exercise-induced asthma (EIA): a constriction of air passages in the tracheobronchial tree of the lungs experienced during exercise. Symptoms include: breathlessness, coughing, and wheezing.

extensor mechanism: the complex structure of muscles, ligaments, and tendons that stabilizes the patella and extends the knee.

fascia: an outer layer of fibrous connective tissue surrounding the muscle.

fats: substances made up of lipids and fatty acids. Certain fats are important for body function. However, the intake of excess fats is associated with cardiovascular diseases.

femur: the bone in the thigh. It is the longest and biggest bone in the human body.

fibrocartilaginous: composed of fibers and cartilages.

fibula: the smaller of the two bones of the leg just below the knee and above the ankle.

flat foot (pes planus): a common condition where the arch of the foot is flat.

follicle stimulating hormone (FSH): a hormone secreted by the brain that stimulates maturation of the follicle in the ovary and promotes the synthesis of sperm in males.

glucose: a simple sugar molecule found naturally in food such as fruits. It is the major source of energy in the cell.

glycogen: a compound made from glucose. It is the major form of stored energy in animal cells, especially in the liver.

glycogen loading: the process by which an athlete loads his cells with excess glycogen by exercising heavily several days before the day of the event and eating large amounts of carbohydrates followed by rest the day before the event. This method stimulates the body to synthesize and store glycogen. In this manner, the athlete has a larger than normal amount of stored glycogen for utilization during the event.

glycolysis: an enzymatic process involving the breakdown of glycogen into simple sugars such as glucose. It is sugars that are utilized to produce energy for the various cellular functions.

gonadotropin hormone: a hormone released by the brain that stimulates the function of the testes and ovaries.

gonadotropin releasing hormone: a hormone secreted by the brain that simulates release of several hormones from the brain, such as gonadotropin hormone, luteinizing hormone (LH), and FSH.

growth center: usually refers to the area at the end of the leg bones that increases in length during the growth period.

growth hormones: hormones secreted by the brain that promote all processes involved in growth and development, including protein synthesis.

hamstring: a large muscle in the back of the thigh responsible for flexing the knee.

heat cramps: muscle spasms associated with pain due to excess heat, which results in loss of water and reduced blood flow to the muscle.

heat exhaustion: caused by water depletion of the body. Symptoms include weakness and malaise.

heat stroke: prolonged exposure to heat and sun resulting in dehydration and loss of thermal regulatory function. Symptoms include a sense of impending doom, headache, dizziness, confusion, and weakness. This is a serious medical emergency that can cause death.

heart rate: frequency of heart muscle contraction (beats) per minute.

heel spur: a bony projection at the back part of the foot: the calcaneus.

hematocrit: a measure of volume of packed cells in blood as percentage of blood volume. The normal range for men is 43–49% and for women 37–43%.

hematoma: blood accumulation in damaged tissue.

hip pointer: damage to the attachments of abdominal and thigh muscles to the back of the pelvis (iliac crest), a very painful injury.

hydrostatic pressure: amount of force exerted per unit surface area.

hyperinsulinemia: an excess amount of insulin secretion.

hypoglycemia: insufficient levels of sugar in the blood.

hypothalamus: a region in the brain involved in controlling body temperature, sleep, and appetite.

hypoxia: an insufficient concentration of oxygen in tissue.

insulin: an important hormone secreted by the pancreas involved in enhancement of energy storage in the cell, such as removal of glucose from the blood into the cell and formation of glycogen from glucose.

intermetatarsal: in between the metatarsal bones of the foot.

interval training: combining maximal exercise sessions alternating with rest periods.

ischemia: reduced oxygenated blood flow to the tissue.

isokinetics: a special method of exercise where tension develops as the muscle contracts.

isotonics: muscle contraction with constant resistance.

Krebs cycle: a sequence of biochemical reactions that break down sugars, fatty acids, and amino acids into carbon dioxide and water. The Krebs cycle produces ATP (adenosine triphosphate), the energy currency for the body.

lactate (lactic acid): an organic acid produced when muscles perform work in the absence of oxygen (an anaerobic process).

lactate shift: a shift to a higher level of tolerance of the blood lactate level due to endurance training.

ligament: fibrous tissue that connects bones to bones. It is present in joints for strength and stability.

luteinizing hormone (LH): secreted by the brain and stimulates secretion of sex hormones in the ovary and testes.

macrotrauma: destruction of large and visible amounts of tissue due to inappropriate or accidental use of that tissue.

medial: toward the midline.

melatonin: a hormone secreted by the brain (the only hormone produced by the pineal gland) that is involved in gonadotropic hormones, skin pigmentation, and many other important functions.

metabolism: refers to all biochemical processes in the body that are involved in areas such as growth, development, energy production, and repair.

metatarsal: relating to bones of the foot.

microcirculation: refers to the blood flow of smaller blood vessels such as capillaries. This system allows for exchange of oxygen from blood to tissues and removal of the waste products of exercise (e.g., carbon dioxide and lactate) from tissue.

microtrauma: destruction of a few cells at a time due to repetitive movement.

mitochondria: an organelle in the cell specializing in production of ATP (adenosine triphosphate).

motor unit: the smallest functional muscle fiber within a motor neuron.

muscle: specialized elongated cells that have the capability to contract and relax, thus causing movement.

muscle fibers (Type I, II): components of muscle. Muscle fibers are formed by a collection of muscle cells and can specialize in long-lasting endurance, a burst of contractions, or medium activity. Type I refers to long-lasting fibers used in marathon running. Type IIA is defined a sprint-type fiber; Type IIB is in between Types IIA and I.

myelination: a sheath of tissue surrounding nerves acting as an electric insulator.

myoglobin: carrier of oxygen in muscle; a counterpart to hemoglobin as the oxygen carrier in the blood.

navicular: refers to the shape of a boat. Usually, navicular bones refer to boat-shaped bones in the foot and hand.

oblique: somewhere between horizontal and perpendicular.

Osgood-Schlatter disease: when the patellar tendon insertion into the tibia is pulled forcefully, causing a tibial nodule. This disease is found mainly in adolescence and is associated with pain and swelling of the knee.

ossification: formation of bone (mostly calcium deposits called calcification).

osteochondritis dissecans: bone fragment separation in a joint.

osteoporosis: loss of bone density usually associated with older women.

overload principle: a gradual increase in workload which results in greater endurance, power, and muscle size.

oxidation: breakdown of chemicals involving oxygen (oxygen receives an electron from hydrogen). This process usually occurs in the mitochondria, the powerhouse of the cell.

patella: the kneecap.

peritendinitis: inflammation of a tendon sheet usually accompanied by pain and swelling.

pH: the negative logarithm of hydrogen ion concentration (i.e., a measure of hydrogen ion concentration). A pH value of 7.0 is neutral, above 7.0 alkaline, and below 7.0 acidic.

phalanges: bones of the finger or toes.

phosphocreatine phosphate: a small organic compound with high energy that can quickly form adenosine triphosphate (ATP) as a source of energy when needed without going through aerobic or anaerobic systems.

phosphorylation: the addition of phosphate into a compound.

planta fascia: fibrous tissue that supports the bottom of the foot.

plasma: the straw-colored fluid portion of the blood consisting of water, electrolytes, proteins, glucose, and other substances (i.e., the liquid portion of the blood).

plica: folding of the tissue.

posterior: a view from the back, opposite to anterior.

power: work output per unit of time.

pressure (overload) training: to exercise above normal level in frequency, intensity, mode, and duration.

progressive principle: increasing overload gradually in order to avoid fatigue and injury.

proprioception: the ability to sense body part positions in space.

protein: a large naturally occurring compound consisting of many amino acids. Proteins are involved in most cellular functions: enzymes, structure, antibodies, etc.

puberty: the period of life when males and females become capable of reproduction.

quadriceps (muscle): the four components of muscle at the front of the thigh: vastus medialis, vastus lateralis, vastus intermedius, and rectus femoris.

respiratory system: breathing system.

sacrum: the backbone area of the pelvis.

serum: the remaining liquid after blood clots. When blood clots, it separates the solid components (e.g., blood cells, platelets, and clotting factors) from the remaining fluid called serum.

shin splint: tendinitis (inflammation) of the tibial area of the leg.

shock: collapse and sudden inability of the cardiovascular system to provide enough blood circulation to the body.

specificity (of training) principle: a training model which emphasizes that training must resemble the sporting activity for which the athlete is training.

splint: a mechanical device used to immobilize a part of the body.

sprain: injury to a ligament.

starch: the main storage food in plants. It consists of long chains of glucose molecules. The counterpart to starch in animals is glycogen.

static stretching: stretching a muscle to a position of slight discomfort and holding it at that position for a period of time.

steroid hormones: natural hormones in the body such as androgens and estrogens involved in sex characteristics and other important functions.

steroids: chemicals that share common structure with the steroid hormones.

strain: overstretching or tearing of a muscle or a tendon.

strength (muscular): the maximal tension (force) generated by the specific muscle group.

stress fracture: when a bone is subjected to repeated and frequent stress, like running on a hard pavement, it causes microfracture of the bone associated with a low level of pain.

stroke volume: blood volume ejected per heart beat.

subluxation: partial dislocation.

subscapularis: one of the shoulder bones of the rotator cuff.

synovial (fluid): lubricating fluid in the joints.

talus: the ankle bone.

tarsal bones: bones (seven of them) at the back of the foot.

tendinitis: inflammation of a tendon which, in the context of sports, is due to injury.

tendon: fibrous tough tissue that attaches skeletal muscle to bones.

thermoregulatory system: a structure located in the hypothalamus responsible for regulation of normal body temperature.

tibia: shin bone (the largest of the two adjacent leg bones).

triglycerides: fats that consist of a fatty acid and a compound called glycerol.

turf toe: a sprain of the joint (metatarsophalangeal) of the large toe.

vasoconstriction: narrowing of blood vessels.

vasodilation: expansion of blood vessels.

viscosity: a parameter of fluid characteristics that relates to the ability of fluid solutions to flow easily.

VO_{2max}: maximal oxygen uptake by a person due to an increased level of exercise.

Index